Taproots

UNDERLYING PRINCIPLES
OF MILTON ERICKSON'S
THERAPY AND HYPNOSIS

A NORTON PROFESSIONAL BOOK

Taproots

UNDERLYING PRINCIPLES
OF MILTON ERICKSON'S
THERAPY AND HYPNOSIS

William Hudson O'Hanlon

W · W · NORTON & COMPANY
NEW YORK · LONDON

Published simultaneously in Canada by Penguin Books Canada Ltd.,
2801 John Street, Markham, Ontario L3R 1B4.
Printed in the United States of America.

Library of Congress Cataloging-in-Publication Data

O'Hanlon, William Hudson.
 Taproots : underlying principles of Milton
Erickson's therapy and hypnosis.

"A Norton professional book."
Bibliography: p.
Includes index.
 1. Erickson, Milton H. 2. Hypnotism — Therapeutic
use. 3. Psychotherapy. I. Title.
RC495.035 1987   616.89'162   86-21853

ISBN 0-393-70031-3

W.W. Norton & Company, Inc.,
500 Fifth Avenue, New York, N.Y. 10110
W.W. Norton & Company, Ltd.,
37 Great Russell Street, London WC1B 3NU

 2 3 4 5 6 7 8 9 0

To Jeffrey K. Zeig, for dragging me up with him.

And to Patricia and Patrick, who are my taproots.

Contents

Preface

An innovative clinician in the fields of hypnosis and therapy, Milton H. Erickson has been the subject of a number of books and articles (see the annotated bibliography for a summary of books by and about Erickson). He himself coauthored several books, and his many papers have been compiled. Nevertheless, a gap has existed in the literature about Erickson's work — we have lacked a practical, unified framework for understanding and using his approaches.

Erickson himself worked for most of his life to discover, use, and teach principles of effective psychotherapy. However, many attempting to learn or master his approach have found his own writings and teaching (via seminars, videotapes and audiotapes) to be inadequate. In his seminars, published articles, and recordings, he roams over much territory, and his wandering, anecdotal style has seemed obtuse, obscure, or overwhelming in its diversity.

Much has been written about his hypnotic approaches and techniques — perhaps too much. Some who approach "Ericksonian" literature or clinical training get the impression that one must be a hypnotist to master Erickson's approach. It is time to dispel this — and many other — misconceptions. Erickson was first and foremost a therapist. As a psychiatrist he helped people resolve their difficulties. In service of this goal, he used many different techniques, approaches, and procedures. Hypnosis was a major tool, but by no means the only approach he used. His work was much more broad-based and flexible than that.

This book offers a unified framework for Ericksonian approaches. It is a book not about hypnosis, but about Erickson's therapeutic procedures. It is an attempt to simplify, but not to oversimplify, the rich diversity of Erickson's work in order to make his procedures accessible to clinicians. My aim is to integrate Erickson's hypnotic and therapeutic approaches and clarify the patterns which connect these two elements of his work. In the desert of the southwest, where both Erickson and I lived for many years, there are plants that send roots down hundreds of feet to tap into underground streams. These are called taproots. In a similar manner, I hope to show that there are underlying principles that give rise to all of Erickson's work, whether hypnotic or nonhypnotic.

Erickson was concerned that his approach might be codified and reified. Therapists learning these reified procedures might try to apply them inappropriately. In so doing, he felt, they would not be responsive to the individual variability and needs of their clients; they would merely imitate Erickson mechanically, not expanding or developing their own procedures and approaches. In his own words (1983), "Develop your own technique. Don't try to use somebody else's technique. . . . Don't try to imitate my voice or my cadence. Just discover your own. Be your own natural self. It's the individual responding to the individual. . . . I've experimented with trying to do something the way somebody else would do it. It's a mess!"

Of course, there are real dangers in codifying any approach. I have attempted in this book to bypass and minimize these pitfalls by offering a set of *patterns* which can be used to generate the kind of interventions that Erickson used. This is not a cookbook; rather, it is a set of approaches, techniques, and ingredients used by a master chef. Each reader can mix and prepare a different dish based on taste and the needs of the hour. Erickson has said, "I don't attempt to structure my psychotherapy except in a vague, general way" (Gordon & Meyers-Anderson, 1981, p. 17).

A number of years ago I started a private practice. As anyone who has ever done so knows, one has a lot of time on one's hands when first starting a practice. I decided to use my spare time to review everything that was written at that time on the work of Milton Erickson, with whom I spent some time in 1977. Erickson's work has mystified many people and I was one of them. I finished my time studying with him more confused than when I started. Although I had studied for several years with Bandler and Grinder and read a number of Erickson's articles, what he demonstrated and talked about was not clear to me. I resolved that I would master and understand Erickson's way of working. What emerged for me during my period of intensive study was a set of patterns that ran through Erickson's work. Over the years since then, I have refined and elaborated the patterns, but I find that they still suffice as a minimal framework for conceptualizing Erickson's work. I call these patterns the "generic patterns" in Erickson's work—"generic" because I have tried to be as descriptive and as atheoretical as possible. One of the difficulties with understanding Erickson's work has been that most analyses are based on theoretical notions that the authors bring to their study of this master clinician. They end up putting Erickson's work into a "Procrustean bed" of their favorite theories and explanations of how people change and what therapy is all about. I have tried to avoid this by being descriptive and providing at most descriptive abstractions. Rather than speculating about Erickson's motivations or purposes, I attempt to provide a model for making sense of and reproducing his therapeutic techniques. I have checked my abstractions against Erickson's work and found them to be accurate. Of course, Erickson, being the creative therapist he was, refuses to be totally captured by any description. This framework serves the purpose of providing a parsimonious model for understanding and reproducing Erickson's work.

The patterns given here can be used to understand and gain access to Erickson's work. The main purpose of the book, however, is to offer therapists some of the powerful tools and approaches Erickson used so that they can more effectively assist their clients to change. If it makes that kind of contribution to the reader, I will be satisfied.

ACKNOWLEDGMENTS

The author acknowledges the help of friends and colleagues who read the manuscript and offered their critical comments. These include Bob Britchford, Frank Butler, Pat Hudson, Sandy Kutler, and Bill and Becky Minier. Additionally, thanks go to Susan Barrows for having faith in my ability to write this and her use of Barrows' razor to produce a clear final product. Finally, an acknowledgment to Milton Erickson, who confused me so much that I decided to go out and figure it out for myself.

Taproots

UNDERLYING PRINCIPLES
OF MILTON ERICKSON'S
THERAPY AND HYPNOSIS

1. Groundwork: Introduction to Erickson's Work

In 1973, I was working at Matthews Art Gallery at Arizona State University. One day, an old gentleman in a wheelchair, accompanied by his wife and daughter, came to the gallery to buy some Seri ironwood carvings. After he left, a colleague at the gallery asked me if I knew who the old gentleman was, and when I said I didn't, she showed me an article about him that was in that week's issue of *Time* magazine ("Svengali in Arizona," October 22, 1973). This was my introduction to Milton Erickson.

A case of Erickson's reported in that article piqued my interest. The case involved a young woman who was depressed. She was very ashamed, she reluctantly admitted, about being so hideous looking. She had a small gap in her front teeth that she thought disfigured her, and as she saw no prospect of getting married and having children, she had lost her will to live. She was planning to commit suicide, but thought she ought to give psychotherapy a chance first. Erickson discovered that she had some money saved and, observing her unkempt appearance, told her to go to a certain clothing store and buy some new outfits. He also told her to go to a certain beauty shop where she was to get a new hairstyle and get instructions in makeup and hygiene. Finally, he told her that she was to practice squirting water through that gap in her teeth while she was in the shower until she could squirt it with accuracy at a distance of seven or eight feet.

Because of some answers the woman had made to his many questions, Erickson had some idea that a certain young man at work was attracted to this young woman. When she would go to the drinking fountain, the young man would invariably show up there at the same time. She, however, did not appreciate his attraction and would just as invariably beat a hasty retreat to her desk and bury her face in her work. Erickson got her to agree, after several sessions, to dress up in her nicest new clothes, fix her hair and makeup and go to work. When the young man showed up at the drinking fountain, she was to get a mouth full of water and squirt it at him through the gap in her teeth. She was to take one step towards him, then turn around and "run like hell!"

The woman was initially reluctant to carry out this assignment, until Erickson reminded her that she did not seem to have one good memory and that, as long as she was planning to die, she ought to die with at least one good memory. She did follow through and to her amazement the young man ran after her, caught her, spun her around and kissed her. The next day he met her at the drinking fountain with a water pistol, she answered with a squirt, and there began a flirtation that ended in a date. She came out of the depression, formed new relationships, and ultimately got married. This was certainly a different approach than I was learning in my psychology courses at the university! It seemed outrageous, yet it seemed to make sense in some ways and it had reportedly worked well. I went out and bought Jay Haley's book on Erickson's work (Haley, 1973), and from then on I was hooked.

It took me some years to screw up the courage to contact Erickson about training with him. In the meantime I had completed my undergraduate degree and worked briefly as a gardener. When I finally contacted him, I had returned to school to seek a master's degree. I wrote a letter telling him that over the years I had come up with various schemes to justify my request for a visit. For example, I thought someone should write an article on his work for *Psychology Today*, or perhaps I would try my hand at writing his biography, as his life story is quite fascinating; I also thought I might barter with him, trading my gardening skills for his teaching. After all was said and done, I wrote, I really just wanted to come and meet him and his wife.

I happened to be away for the weekend shortly after that, and when I returned my roommate told me that the strangest man had called early each morning. He asked for the "O'Hanlon Gardening Service." Upon being told that I was not home, he hung up, leaving no message.

The next morning, right on cue, the phone rang and it was the "strange man" asking for the O'Hanlon Gardening Service. I told him that this was Bill O'Hanlon and he said, "Don't you think you ought to survey the territory before you decide to take the job?" I asked if this was Dr. Erickson, and when he replied in the affirmative I told him that I thought I should indeed survey the territory. We made an appointment for the next week.

When I arrived, dressed in my best clothes, he and his wife, Betty, showed me around the house and let me see some scrapbooks they had. Then Erickson had me take him out to the garden. I had thought that the bit about the gardening service was just a metaphor. It certainly may have been a metaphor, but I soon learned that it was not *just* a metaphor. He told me that he wanted me to weed the "nut grass" out of the roses. I was very uncomfortable with this request, as I had on some nice clothes, but I was too intimidated to protest. I worked in his garden on a regular basis for some time after that and occasionally sat in on a session. I often left feeling more confused than ever about what he had been doing. Was he doing therapy as he sat and talked to me as I gardened?

He always answered questions about what he wanted done in the garden in a straightforward way, but he was nowhere near as enlightening when I asked a question about therapy. So I ended this time with Erickson more confused than when I started. I vowed that I would someday figure out his approach. I had the sense, as Jay Haley has said, that if I only understood more of what Erickson was saying, my therapy would improve greatly. Here then are the results of my quest and the fruits of my labors.

ROOTS OF AN
INNOVATIVE PSYCHIATRIST

Milton Erickson was trained as a psychiatrist and a psychologist, completing his training in 1929. He had an early interest in hypnosis that was stimulated by seeing the behavioral psychologist Clark Hull do a demonstration. Erickson subsequently explored hypnosis both experimentally and clinically. His initial professional positions were with state asylums (mental hospitals). It was here that many of the experiments that led him to develop his innovative approaches were conducted. At that time there were not many successful approaches and techniques for doing therapy with severely disturbed individuals. The psychotropic drugs that later became popular as management tools for these people were not yet available. So, out of necessity, Erickson developed many innovative approaches to managing and treating these disorders. Hypnosis was his primary, but by no means his only, tool. After a time, his writings show that he started to generalize from the hypnotic experiments, experiences, and techniques into a broader "hypnotic" approach to psychotherapy. He used his mastery of hypnotic communication skills and interpersonal influence in therapy that used no formal trance.

The influence of this early hypnotic practice is apparent throughout Erickson's later work. It appears both in the specific techniques and distinguishing features of his mature work and in the generic patterns and underlying principles. Evidence of this influence is abundant throughout the present book. In fact, a central premise of this work is that *there is an underlying unity to Erickson's hypnosis and his therapy work.*

DISTINGUISHING CHARACTERISTICS:
BASIC PRINCIPLES

One can discuss the basics of Erickson's approach under the following headings: naturalistic, indirect and directive, responsiveness, utilization, and present and future orientation. Each of these terms refers to a specific principle that typifies Erickson's work, whether hypnotic or therapeutic.

The Naturalistic Orientation

Erickson believed that people have within them the natural abilities to overcome difficulties, to resolve problems, to go into a trance and to have all of the trance phenomena. His approach was to elicit those natural abilities. He was very much opposed to trying to *teach* people things in psychotherapy. "Now, too much has been written and said and done about the reeducation of the neurotic and the psychotic and the maladjusted personality. As if anybody could really tell any one person how to think and how to feel and how to react to any given situation. Everybody reacts differently, according to his own background of personal experience" (Erickson, 1966). Nothing needed to be added from the outside, as all the answers were within. Erickson had a basic view of human beings as capable and of nature as maintaining and supporting health if allowed to. Normal behavior and growth are to be expected; symptoms and pathology are blockages of that natural healthiness. Trance, in his view, was a natural skill or ability, an everyday experience. The therapist's task was to create a context so that patients could gain access to abilities and resources they had not previously been using to resolve their problems.

The other side of this naturalistic coin was that psychotherapy and hypnosis could be carried out in such a way that they appeared to be very natural situations and conversations. Hypnosis did not need to be a formal ritual and the subject did not need to be aware that the trance induction had begun or was happening. The same was true of the therapy. Erickson often told anecdotes and gave assignments that were not easily recognized as therapeutic interventions. Therapy could be a very natural, nonritualistic process.

Indirect and Directive Orientations

It is often said both that Erickson was directive and that he used indirect techniques and suggestions. This may seem to be a contradiction in terms, but actually is not. Erickson told this story in a teaching seminar:

I was returning from high school one day and a runaway horse with a bridle on sped past a group of us into a farmer's yard . . . looking for a drink of water. The horse was perspiring heavily. And the farmer didn't recognize it, so we cornered it. I hopped on the horse's back . . . since it had a bridle on, I took hold of the rein and said, "Giddy-up" . . . headed for the highway. I knew the horse would turn in the right direction . . . I didn't know what the right direction was. And the horse trotted and galloped along. Now and then he would forget he was on the highway and start into a field. So I would pull on him a bit and call his attention to the fact that the highway was where he was supposed to be. And finally about four miles from where I had boarded him he turned into a farm yard and the farmer said, "So that's how that critter came back. Where did you find him?"

I said, "About four miles from here."
"How did you know he should come here?"
I said, "I didn't know . . . the horse knew. All I did was keep
his attention on the road."
. . . I think that's the way you do psychotherapy. (Gordon
& Meyers-Anderson, 1981, p. 6)

Erickson *was* very directive in getting people to do things
and in blocking old patterns that maintained the symptom.
He did not want to ever tell people how to live or how they
should handle life in general. He thought this was wrong. "As
if anybody could really tell any one person how to think and
how to feel and how to react in any given situation!" He gave
assignments or suggestions that provided for just enough
loosening of rigidities for the person to discover other ways
of thinking and behaving that would eliminate the symptom.
He gave suggestions and directions that allowed patients to
find their own meanings and ways to solve their own problems.

Erickson was very directive in dealing with symptoms and
very indirect in matters pertaining to the way people would
live their lives after the symptom was resolved or even how,
specifically, they would resolve the symptom. "Too many
hypnotherapists take you out to dinner and then tell you what
to order. I take a patient out to dinner and I say, 'You give
your order.' The patient makes his own selection of the food
he wants. He is not hindered by my instructions, which would
only obstruct and obscure his inner processes" (Erickson, in
Rossi, 1980).

Responsiveness

Although a common concern for most hypnotists, hypnotiz-
ability was not a topic Erickson discussed very much. Moreover, Erickson was able to achieve results with people whom

most therapists or hypnotists might have found extremely difficult, if not impossible, to treat successfully. Both phenomena
are related to the "responsiveness" view that Erickson seemed
to hold. People are not set as they express themselves currently. They are able to respond to different stimuli with
different responses. Instead of attributing unworkability to
rigid personality characteristics, Erickson would take it upon
himself to learn the individual's patterns of behavior and
response. He would then utilize these patterns in service of
change, rather than treating them as blocks.

Utilization Orientation

Most therapists and hypnotists have preconditions for their
patients. Erickson seemed to have few or no expectations or
prerequisites for what constituted a workable situation in
hypnosis and therapy. Whatever the patient presented was
utilized. Erickson used rigid beliefs, behaviors, demands, and
characteristics so that they not only did not interfere with the
desired results, but even facilitated the therapy.

The things that Erickson often utilized in treatment included: presenting problems and symptoms, rigid beliefs and
delusions, and rigid behavior patterns. A few examples will
illustrate each type of utilization.

*Erickson utilized the symptom in a case in which a woman's
in-laws were constantly dropping in to visit and staying longer
than she wanted them to stay. She developed an ulcer. Erickson told her that while her ulcer incapacitated her at work,
at church, in her social relationships, and with her family, it
was really just her in-laws who gave her "a pain in the belly."
She should learn to use her ulcer in the situation where she
needed it and where it could do her some good. The woman
liked this idea. The next few times her in-laws came to visit,
she drank a glass of milk hurriedly and, after a few minutes*

*of visiting, vomited. Since she was ill, she could not be ex-
pected to clean up, so the in-laws had to mop the floor. They
quit visiting so often and began to call before coming. If she
did not want them to visit, she would mention that her ulcer
had been acting up. If she did want them to visit and they
were overstaying their welcome, she would start to massage
her stomach and look as if she were in pain. They would quickly beat a retreat. After some time, the ulcer healed (Haley,
1985, Vol. 1, pp. 45–46).*

In a case illustrating the use of the patient's rigid beliefs
and delusions to further therapy, Erickson approached a man
at the state hospital who claimed to be Jesus Christ and told
him that he understood the patient had had experience as a
carpenter. Knowing that Jesus did indeed help his father,
Joseph, who was a carpenter, the man could only reply that
he had. Erickson said that he also understood that the patient
wanted to be of service to his fellow man. To this, the patient
also answered in the affirmative. Erickson then informed him
that the hospital needed help building some bookcases and
asked for his cooperation in the matter. The patient agreed
and was able to start participating in constructive behavior
rather than continuing his symptomatic behavior (Haley, 1973,
p. 28).

An example of using rigid behavior in the service of a
therapeutic goal occurred when a woman sought therapy with
Erickson, reporting that she had been unsuccessful in her past
efforts at therapy. She had a compulsive need to comment
on the details of her environment. Even as she gave this brief
statement, she carried on an endless and uninterruptable
stream of comments on the immediate environment. Erickson
began making movements, like cleaning his glasses and moving his desk blotter. She immediately commented on each of
these actions. He then gradually slowed and hesitated in his

movements and she began to wait for him in her comments. As the session went on, she relied more and more on Erickson's actions to structure her rate of speech. After some time, he was able to offer interjections of his own which led to a trance induction and a successful therapeutic relationship (Rossi, 1980, Vol. 1, pp. 179–181).

Pattern intervention is discussed in more detail in Chapter 2. The main point here is that there are no prerequisites for the presentation, personality, behavior, beliefs, etc., that the person brings to the therapist or the hypnotist. Whatever the person presents is taken to be the starting point for successful psychotherapy and is used, if possible, in service of the desired goal.

Present and Future Orientation

Perhaps Erickson was not the first therapist to bring a more here-and-now, present orientation to psychotherapy, in contradistinction to the historical orientation of analytic and psychodynamic orientations. But he almost certainly was the first to bring a *future* orientation to psychotherapy. He was not interested in "psychological archeology" and attempted to orient people away from the past into the present and the future, where they could deal with difficulties more adequately. "Psychotherapy," he wrote, "is sought not primarily for enlightenment about the unchangeable past but because of dissatisfaction with the present and a desire to better the future" (in Watzlawick, Weakland, & Fisch, 1974, p. ix). "The past cannot be changed," he said, "only one's views and interpretations of it, and even these change with the passage of time. Hence, at best, views and interpretations of the past are of importance only when they stultify the person into a rigidity. Life is lived in the present for the morrow. Hence, psychotherapy is properly oriented about life today in preparation for tomorrow, next month, next year, the future, which in itself will compel many changes in the functioning of the person at all levels of his behavior" (in Beahrs, 1971, p. 74).

In a sense, one could say that Erickson was not *problem*-oriented, but *solution*-oriented. He did not favor looking back at the past to see the origins of the problem or the learned limitations of the person. He was oriented towards solutions and strengths that existed for the person in the present or that could be developed and used in the future.

DISTINGUISHING CHARACTERISTICS: THERAPIST STANCES

Flexibility

> Each person is an individual. Hence, psychotherapy should be formulated to meet the uniqueness of the individual's needs, rather than tailoring the person to fit the Procrustean bed of a hypothetical theory of human behavior. (Erickson, 1979)

Erickson stressed the need for therapists to be flexible, and his work showed evidence of the importance of flexibility in making hypotheses and in acting therapeutically.

Erickson saw no point in becoming wedded to one's hypothesis. Consider that, despite almost a century of experimental inquiry into the matter, there is still very little agreement about the causes of human behavior and experience. Many profess to know the rhyme and reason to human behavior. Their ideological opponents, however, argue just as persuasively and vociferously for opposing explanations and conceptualizations. Given our present state of knowledge, there seems to be no certainty in this realm of etiology.

An appropriate stance for the therapist, therefore, is one that leaves room for alternate explanations, meanings, and motivations for human behavior and experience. It has been suggested that, given the current state of understanding in this field, perhaps a better criterion than "true/false" for evaluating hypotheses in a clinical setting would be "more useful/less useful" (Bandler & Grinder, 1975).

In his early hypnotic studies, Erickson discovered the importance of flexibility in the therapist's behavior. He found that if he changed his behavior and communication, it had a marked effect on his subjects' experiences. He discovered that sometimes slight changes in the therapist's or hypnotist's words, behavior, and communications could lead to dramatic alterations in the experience of trance subjects. He extended this orientation to his therapeutic work. If what he was doing was not eliciting the desired response, Erickson would do something else. He was not bound by any theory in making these changes — just by a sense of curiosity and flexibility combined with a keen sense of observation. As Haley (1973, p. 203) wrote, "Erickson has no set method. His approach is oriented to the particular person and his situation, and he feels that only with experience can one know what to do with a particular child. A part of his success is determined by his tenacity when working with a patient. If one procedure doesn't work, he tries others until one does."

Observation

> When you want to find things out about your patients, observe. Observe their behavior. (Erickson, in Rosen, 1982)

> Erickson was a lucid naturalist who felt no need to go much beyond the sense observations of what was immediately present. (Rossi, Ryan, & Sharp, 1983)

Erickson often stressed to his students the importance of observation. In line with the emphasis on flexibility in hypothesizing, he also stressed that the therapist does not know for certain the meaning of the things he observes. He emphasized the use of all the therapist's sensory modalities, especially watching and listening, in the search for clues to effective therapy and to how therapy was working. The patient's language, changes in vocal dynamics, alterations in muscle tonus and gestures were some of the things he mentioned as important to observe. He delighted in recounting the story of the time he had asked his medical students to give him an objective description of the man who stood before them. He asked the man to come in and stand sideways so that one half of the students could see one side and the other half the other side. When the first group proclaimed that the man had blue eyes, the second group protested that the man's eyes were brown. Neither was correct, Erickson demonstrated, as he asked the man to reenter the room and show that he had one blue eye and one brown eye. Observe! was the message and don't go beyond the facts.

Erickson's sensitivity to subtleties in communication was far beyond most people's. He may have developed his unusual powers of observation while he was paralyzed with polio. At that time one of his pastimes was to attend to verbal and nonverbal communications, as there was not much else to engage his inquiring mind while other family members went about their daily business. Erickson once told me about a psychiatrist who came to him and was talking about his ex-wife. The man claimed that for professional reasons he did not want to tell Erickson his ex-wife's name, but he kept dropping hints to the contrary. During the session, Erickson got a nagging sense of wanting to call an acquaintance of his. He interrupted the session to call this woman and told her that even though her name was Kathy, he had the strangest urge to call her Nancy. As he said this, he looked meaningfully at the psychiatrist, who was listening as Erickson talked on the phone. When Erickson said the name Nancy, the psychiatrist exclaimed that that was his ex-wife's name. The man opened up more after Erickson's discovery of his ex-wife's name. When

I asked Erickson how he knew the name, he replied that his
unconscious must have picked it up. The man had probably
stressed the syllables "nan" and "see" as he was talking to
Erickson. His unconscious, through association with his friend
Kathy, had put the clues together (Erickson, 1977).

Haley relates another story about Erickson's keen powers
of observation. A physician who was a resident under Erickson
told Haley that one day Erickson met the man's wife walking
on the hospital grounds. After exchanging amenities with her,
he remarked that she was obviously pregnant. She was shocked
that he would say so, as she had just come from the gynecol-
ogist's office, where she had found out that she was pregnant.
Erickson told her that he had observed the change in colora-
tion on her forehead (called "chloasma") that he had seen before on pregnant women (Haley, 1982, p. 13).

If the therapist is to have a flexible, responsive orientation,
it is obviously important to be able to notice when the desired
response has occurred. Most of us will never develop Erickson's powers of observation, and we probably do not need to
for most situations that confront us in therapy. The important point here is that an ability to observe was an important
part of Erickson's orientation. The question of *what* to observe
is also important and will be discussed in future chapters.

Assumptions to be Avoided

There are some assumptions that therapists have tradition-
ally held which Erickson challenged. His views about these
assumptions are outlined below.

On the necessity of knowing the cause
of a problem to resolve it

Erickson did not believe that the therapist or the client had
to know the cause of the symptom or problem in order to

resolve it. "Etiology is a complex matter and not always relevant to getting over a problem" (Erickson, in Haley, 1973, p. 106). Some theorists (e.g., Keeney, 1983, 1985; O'Hanlon & Wilk, 1987; Watzlawick, 1984) have even suggested that one can never know with certainty the cause of any human situation. In any case, Erickson sometimes treated a case successfully without, in his words, "inquiring when it started, nor how it started, nor what caused it" (in Haley, 1985, Volume 1, p. 29).

On the necessity of insight/awareness for change

Perhaps the most radical departure in Erickson's approach was his deemphasis on and even opposition to the promotion of insight or awareness to precipitate change.

> . . . Many psychotherapists regard as almost axiomatic that therapy is contingent on making the unconscious conscious. When thought is given to the immeasurable role the unconscious plays in the total experiential life of a person from infancy on, whether awake or asleep, there can be little expectation of doing more than making some small parts of it conscious. Furthermore, the unconscious as such, not as transformed into the conscious, constitutes an essential part of psychological functioning. (Erickson, in Rossi, 1980, Vol. 4, p. 246)

On the necessity of having a coherent theory and general hypotheses

Erickson believed that preconceptions about patients hampered the therapist, so he strove to have no particular theory or general hypotheses about problems. He preferred instead to take each case as it came, hypothesizing on matters for each particular client.

On the immutability of character/ personality

> Your patient is one person today, quite another person to-
> morrow, and still another person next week, next month,
> next year. Five years from now, ten and twenty years from
> now, he is yet another person. We all have a certain gen-
> eral background, that is true, but we are different persons
> each day that we live. (Erickson, in Rossi, Ryan, & Sharp,
> 1983, p. 3)

Erickson seemed to operate for the most part as if people
have the possibility of changing their behavior, the expression
of their personality, and other aspects of themselves. Unlike
other practitioners, who believe that personality is fixed geneti-
cally or at a very young age, Erickson seemed to take the
pragmatic stance that personality (or at least personality expression) is very mutable. His therapy was usually based on
the assumption that there were alternative aspects of the
personality that could be brought forth and used for the person's benefit.

On the function and origin of symptoms

A very common idea of therapists, across many persuasions,
theories and schools, is that symptoms arise because they serve
functions. They believe that symptoms not only arise to serve
functions, but also continue to serve some function for the
person (e.g., intrapsychic relief of anxiety) or their social system
(e.g., family); otherwise, they contend, they would not continue. Because Erickson sometimes just worked for symptom
relief, with no discussion or resolution of the underlying problem or function, he came to hold a different view. Perhaps
problems arose for functional reasons, but after a time they

might stop serving that function; they might continue just because human beings are so patterned. I have found in teaching therapists Erickson's approach that this concept is very difficult for most of them to incorporate. Even Jay Haley, Erickson's longtime student and popularizer, had a difficult time with this concept when he first started conversing with Erickson in the 1950s. Haley asked Erickson about a particular case and when Erickson made suggestions that would "merely" resolve the symptom, Haley objected on the grounds that the symptom surely served some purpose. Erickson replied, "Your assumption is that it served other purposes. Have you ever thought about symptomatology wearing out in serving purposes and becoming a habitual pattern?" (Haley, 1985, Volume 1, p. 15)

In a similar manner, Erickson did not hold the view that symptoms are always expressions of underlying problems or past trauma. "I think that the vast majority of habits developed by people tend to be habits based on habitual patterns of response, and so they are not necessarily symptomatic of deep traumatic experiences" (Erickson, in Rossi & Ryan, 1985, p. 21).

The Burden of Responsibility for Results in Therapy

In Erickson's view, both the therapist and the client have roles in obtaining results in therapy.

The therapist's responsibility is to create a climate, an atmosphere for change. He does this by creating an atmosphere of expectancy for success (through his words and actions) and by utilizing and incorporating the patient's objections, style, and "resistance" into the treatment. "In psychotherapy you change no one. People change themselves. You create circumstances under which an individual can respond spontaneously and change. And that's all you do. The rest is up to them" (Erickson, in Ritterman, 1985, p. 69).

The client's responsibility is to *do* something, either experientially or behaviorally or both. "The thing to do," Erickson said, "is to get your patient, any way you wish, any way you can, to do something. . . . It is the patient who does the therapy. The therapist only furnishes the climate, the weather. That's all. The patient has to do all the work" (Erickson, in Zeig, 1980, pp. 143, 148).

Erickson was very focused on getting people to carry out some activity, whether internal (experiential) or external (behavioral). His therapy was oriented towards initiating the activity. He used the analogy of the starting pistol at the race: The therapist merely initiates the race by firing the starting pistol; it is the patient who must actually run and win the race (Rossi, Ryan, & Sharp, 1983, pp. 102–103).

Generic
Patterns

2. Pattern Intervention

> ... maladies, whether psychogenic or organic, followed
> definite patterns of some sort, particularly in the field
> of psychogenic disorders; that a disruption of this pattern
> could be a most therapeutic measure; and that it often
> mattered little how small the disruption was, if intro-
> duced early enough ...
>
> Erickson, in Rossi, 1980, Vol. 4, p. 254

Erickson often made the observation that people's behavior
and thinking are rigidly patterned, but, instead of concluding
that because they are rigid they will never change (as many
therapies do), he viewed patterns as changeable. His hypnosis
and therapy showed three major approaches to intervening
in patterns: (1) the utilization of current patterns in service
of change; (2) alteration or blocking of current patterns; and
(3) establishing new patterns.

UTILIZATION OF CURRENT PATTERNS

One of the cornerstones of Erickson's approach was the
acceptance and utilization of the patient's patterns of behavior
and experience (and of social and family patterns of interaction
as well). This involved not merely accepting nonjudgmentally
what the patient presented, but actively discovering and using
these patterns in the service of change. At various times and
various places, Erickson stressed the utilization of:

a) The patient's language
b) The patient's interests and motivations
c) The patient's beliefs and frames of reference
d) The patient's behavior
e) The patient's symptom(s)
f) The patient's resistance.

Utilizing the Patient's Language

Too often psychotherapists try to deal with their patients by using their doctoral degree language, trying to explain the ego, superego, and the id, conscious and unconscious, and the patient doesn't know whether you're talking about corn, potatoes or hash. Therefore, you try to use the language of the patient. (Erickson, in Gordon & Meyers-Anderson, 1981, p. 49)

Perhaps the best-known example of Erickson's use of the patient's language is the case of the state hospital patient who came under Erickson's care and spoke only "schizophrenese" or "word salad." The man spoke English, but uttered only meaningless (to others) phrases like " . . . bucket of sand, bucket of lard, fat's in the fire, had a flat tire. . . . " He had been in the hospital for over nine years, and although he seemed to be attempting to communicate with others, no one had as yet been able to understand him. He had arrived at the hospital without identification, no history had been elicited, and no therapy had been provided. When Erickson inherited the case, he sent a stenographer to sit at a desk near the man and surreptitiously record the man's utterances. After these were transcribed, Erickson studied them closely, but could discern no meaningful communications in them. He decided, therefore, that he would speak "word salad" and communicate to the patient in his own language. He introduced himself to the man, and when the man uttered some word salad in response,

Erickson responded with some word salad, uttered in a sincere tone. At first the patient seemed skeptical, but he soon began carrying on long conversations with Erickson in word salad. He even started interspersing meaningful utterances in his word salad, and over time the percentage of sensible communications increased. Gradually Erickson obtained a history, provided therapy, and facilitated the man's release from the hospital (Gordon & Meyers-Anderson, 1981, pp. 52–53; Rossi, 1980, Vol. 4, pp. 213–215).

Most of the time, Erickson did not have to go to such lengths to use the patient's language, of course. He spoke to people using their words and at a level they could understand.

Utilizing the Patient's Interests and Motivations

> She has a very strong desire to do good work. She is strong there, so I'm using that motivation to deal with the place where she is weak—her airplane phobia. (Erickson, in Erickson & Rossi, 1979, p. 333)

In keeping with his naturalistic principle, Erickson tried to discover and use his patients' interests and motivation. Rather than to worry about their lack of motivation, he would find out what they were interested in and what they were motivated to do and then link the therapy to that motivation. A case example might best illustrate this principle.

A policeman who had retired for medical reasons sought Erickson's help after his doctor had vetoed the policeman's idea of running to get back in shape. The doctor had said that running would be too risky, considering the man's emphysema, his high blood pressure, his gross obesity, his smoking and his drinking. The most he could do was to walk. He re-

ferred the ex-policeman to Erickson as he considered it a psy-chiatric problem. Erickson found out that the man lived alone, did all his own cooking, and shopped for his food, as well as his liquor and cigarettes, at the corner store just down from his second-floor apartment. Erickson recommended that the man buy his cigarettes only one pack at a time and walk across town to get each pack. He also told him to find a grocery store at least a half mile away and buy only enough for each meal while he was shopping there. As for drinking, he recommended that the man could drink all he wanted, provided he walked a mile for that first drink and at least a mile for each single drink thereafter. Erickson commented, "Now, I didn't take food away from him. I didn't take tobacco away. I didn't take liquor away. I gave him the opportunity to walk" (Rosen, 1982, pp. 149–150).

In a case of Zeig's (1985, p. 68) a woman was going to sell her business, and Zeig thought this would be disadvantageous for her in the long run. He consulted Erickson, who had seen the woman and her family in therapy previously. Erickson advised Zeig to tell the woman to keep the business because it would set a good example for her children. Zeig reported that the ploy worked, as being a good model for her children was very important to the woman.

Utilizing the Patient's Beliefs and Frames of Reference

In other words, you try to accept the patient's ideas no mat-ter what they are, and then you try to direct them. (Erick-son, in Erickson & Rossi, 1981, p. 13)

There is a tale that illustrates this principle very well. It concerns a prince in ancient times who became convinced that he was a chicken. He shed all his clothes and refused to eat anything but corn off the ground, much to the consternation of his father, the king. The king brought great physicians and wise men from near and far to try to help his poor son, but alas, none succeeded in convincing the prince he was not a chicken nor in getting him to give up his unusual behavior. Finally, a wise man came to the palace and offered to cure the prince. The king was skeptical, as he had already seen so many failures, but gave his permission for the man to try. The wise man asked that he be left alone with the prince. When they were alone, the wise man shed his clothes and joined the prince in eating corn off the floor. The prince looked at the wise man suspiciously and challenged him, asking who he was. The wise man answered that he was a chicken and went on eating corn. He then asked the prince who he was and the prince replied that he too was a chicken. After a time the prince accepted the wise man as his equal. One day the wise man got up and put on some clothing. The prince was shocked and protested that chickens do not wear clothes. The wise man merely replied that he was a chicken and he was wearing clothes, so obviously chickens do wear clothes. After a time the prince too began to wear some clothes. A while later, the wise man started to eat some of the "human" food that was brought to them every day. Again the prince protested and again the reply was given that he, the wise man, was a chicken and was eating that food, so obviously chickens can eat "human" food. In time, the wise man started walking upright and gave the same rationale for it when the prince protested. Gradually, the prince was led back to being a chicken who acted very much like a man and the delusion passed.

The beliefs the patient brings to therapy are to be utilized in the service of the changes he or she would like to make. Erickson did not often try to directly correct patients' irrational beliefs. Instead, he used those beliefs to lead patients out of their problems.

A woman too embarrassed to telephone wrote to Erickson requesting an appointment. When she finally appeared for her appointment, she related an incident which occurred while she was in a college classroom. She was writing on the blackboard when she loudly passed flatus. She was so embarrassed that she ran from the classroom and stayed in her apartment for six months, venturing out only at night for groceries. Erickson discovered that she was very religious and he accused her of being irreligious and blasphemous. She was indignant in her denial of these charges. Erickson asked her if she thought God made her in his image. She replied that He did. Then he asked her if she thought that any human engineer could design a valve that opened downward and held in liquids and solids while letting only gas through. She thought it was unlikely. Erickson asserted that that was just what God had done when he made her anus and that she really ought to learn to appreciate His marvelous handiwork. He said he would help her by telling her to go home and cook herself a big pot of beans (they're called "whistleberries" in the Navy, he said) and practice making big ones, little ones, loud ones and soft ones. She agreed to do the task and eventually returned to school (Rosen, 1982, pp. 151–152).

A final example of utilizing the patient's beliefs and frames of reference was Erickson's treatment of a farmworker who thought he was worthless. Erickson was attempting to get Harold to take better care of himself, to eat more appropriately, and to move out of his rundown shack and into better quarters. Harold was reluctant to follow this advice until Erickson started talking about how a tractor was only a machine meant to do farm work. Harold readily understood this analogy. Erickson pointed out that a farm machine should be properly cared for or it ceased being useful. He told Harold in great detail what the proper care of farm machinery involved. With this new framework Harold was willing to make the changes

Erickson suggested in his hygiene and his living conditions
(Haley, 1973, p. 128).

Utilizing the Patient's Behavior

> In brief, whatever the behavior manifested by the subjects,
> it should be accepted and regarded as grist for the mill.
> (Erickson, in Rossi, 1980, Vol. 1, p. 158)

> By naturalistic approach is meant the acceptance and uti-
> lization of the situation encountered without endeavoring
> to psychologically restructure it. In so doing, the present-
> ing behavior becomes a definite aid and an actual part in
> inducing a trance, rather than a possible hindrance. (Erick-
> son, in Rossi, 1980, Vol. 1, p. 168)

A man sought therapy from Erickson, but explained that
he couldn't sit down or lie down and talk about his problems.
He had already been dismissed from several psychiatrists'
offices for being uncooperative and unworkable. He explained
that he was too anxious to sit or lie still and that being in a
psychiatrist's office made the anxiety worse. Erickson asked
the man if he would be willing to continue to pace in the office
as he was currently doing. The man affirmed that he would
and said that pacing was the only way he could stay in the
office at all. Erickson asked the man if he would mind if
Erickson directed his pacing. The man was a bit bewildered
by the request, but he again agreed. Erickson spent some time
directing the man in his pacing and gradually slowed his rate
of speaking. The man responded by pacing more slowly and
gradually coming to wait for Erickson's directions before he
walked. After about 45 minutes, the man, by this time used
to following Erickson's directives, responded to Erickson's
direct suggestion to sit down and go deeply into trance (Rossi,
1980, Vol. 1, pp. 181–182).

Utilizing the Patient's Symptom(s)

> By using the patient's own patterns of response and behavior, including those of their actual illness, one may effect therapy more promptly and satisfactorily, with resistance to therapy greatly obviated and acceptance of therapy facilitated. (Erickson, in Rossi, 1980, Vol. 4, p. 348)

The case of the young woman with the gap in her teeth discussed in the first chapter is an example of using symptoms, in this case the gap in her teeth and her suicidal ideation, to facilitate treatment. In this case, both were utilized not only to facilitate but also to directly effect, therapeutic goals. The symptom became the solution under Erickson's guidance. Erickson wrote about this type of utilization in a 1965 paper entitled "The Use of Symptoms as an Integral Part of Hypnotherapy" (Rossi, 1980, Vol. 4, pp. 212–223). With his typically positive outlook, Erickson tended to show great respect for symptoms and the skill that they showed. One could argue that he used every so-called defense mechanism in the service of change. For example, hallucinations are usually viewed as only negative, but Erickson often deliberately induced hallucinations as part of hypnotic treatment. Many therapists are concerned about the phenomenon of symptom substitution (i.e., one symptom replacing another), but Erickson would sometimes deliberately encourage symptom substitution as a means of creating a problem that was easier to solve or that would interfere less in the patient's life.

Utilizing the Patient's Resistance

> One always tries to use whatever the patient brings into the office. If they bring in resistance, be grateful for that resistance. Heap it up in whatever fashion they want you to — really pile it up! (Erickson, in Erickson & Rossi, 1981, p. 16)

Resistances constituting a part of the problem can be utilized by enhancing them and thereby permitting the patient to discover, under guidance, new ways of behavior favorable to recovery. (Erickson, in Rossi, 1980, Vol. 4, p. 48)

When I first drove a car, the key that started the car was inserted with the jagged edge pointing towards the floor of the car. The next car, however, had just the opposite standard, the jagged edge of the key pointed away from the floor. I always thought that the key to the second car was inserted upside down. Some patients seem to have their keys in "upside down," and require an approach that takes into account their oppositional response patterns. In a case of a resistant demonstration subject determined not to go into trance, Erickson merely directed the man to stay wider and wider awake, to keep his eyes open, etc. Since he was determined to resist Erickson's directives, the man was compelled to comply with the trance induction (Haley, 1963, p. 35).

Matching Current Patterns

Another way in which Erickson utilized current patterns was to match the patterns of behavior and language that patients showed. One of his most notable skills was his ability to quickly gain rapport with people who would not typically be easy to work with in therapy. He was also known for his ability to get people to follow directives that many people might hesitate to follow if they were given by other therapists. One of the ways he achieved both of these effects was by matching his behavior, vocabulary, and ideas to the patient's behavior, experience, and understanding. Matching is accomplished by the therapist's mirroring the patient's physical behaviors and vocabulary. Erickson probably developed and mastered this technique in the context of his hypnotic work. In the hypnotic setting, the effects of such matching on rapport are more obvious than in other communicational settings. The person in trance is usually not moving or talking as much as in ordinary settings, so responses are usually more noticeable. When a hypnotist says or does something which does not match the patient, the response is usually apparent very rapidly in the subject's behavior, in that the subject's trance is disrupted.

Starting by matching patients' behavior and by meeting them at their frame of reference, the therapist or hypnotist can gently or subtly lead the patients in the direction of the desired outcome.

Biorapport

Various anecdotal and scientific sources have reported the phenomenon of rhythmic alignment of people who are affiliated and in rapport. Female roommates' menstrual cycles line up with one another. Psychotherapists and patients tend to move at the same time, use similar gestures, take similar postures, etc. (see Scheflen, 1965). These phenomena can be considered examples of biorapport. This rhythmic biological attunement seems to both indicate and enhance rapport between people. Erickson used this rhythmic matching deliberately to facilitate the development of rapport and to influence patients. Most often mentioned in this type of rapport-building is the matching of breathing patterns. Basically, the therapist aligns the rhythm of his voice, his movements, or his own breathing with the patient's breathing rhythm. Erickson's manuscript on this subject ("Respiratory Rhythm in Trance Induction: The Role of Minimal Sensory Cues in Normal and Trance Behavior," in Rossi, 1980, Vol. 1, pp. 360–365) contains a more detailed account of the use of this procedure. Ernest Rossi, one of Erickson's students and collaborators, has discussed Erickson's use of ultradian rhythms, the cycles of physiological activity and rest that run through the day (Rossi, 1982, 1985).

ALTERING EXISTING PATTERNS

... And then what you need to do is to try to do something
that induces a change in the patient ... any little change,
because the patient wants a change, however small, and he
will accept that as a change. .... He will accept that as a
change and then follow that change and the change will
develop in accord with his own needs. .... It's much like roll-
ing a snowball down a mountainside. It starts out a small
snowball, but as it rolls down it gets larger and larger ... and
it becomes an avalanche that fits to the shape of the moun-
tain. (Erickson, in Gordon & Meyers-Anderson, 1981, pp.
16–17)

Erickson did not really have a formal theory of how problems arise or of psychopathology. The closest he came was
his view of rigid behavior. He observed the rigidity in patients'
beliefs and behavior and considered it pathological. Where
rigidity has been, he seemed to be saying, let there be flexibility. If flexibility were introduced, the pathology would disappear or at least be very diminished in its detrimental effects.
To this end, Erickson often elicited a quite detailed description of the presenting problem from the client and then used
that information to devise an intervention that would alter
some aspect of the symptom complex. This enables the therapist to get some initial influence over the expression of the
symptom. Once the therapist successfully gets the client to
alter one aspect of the symptom, he may be able to alter other
aspects of the symptom. This could ultimately result in the
resolution of the presenting problem. Another aspect of this
type of intervention is that if the client is able to change one
part of a symptom previously experienced as a rigid unalter-
able "thing," he might more easily accept the idea that change
is possible.

If the term "symptom" is used as shorthand for "undesired
behavior or experience which the client is seeking to eliminate," there are numerous parameters of the symptom's oc-

currence which can be considered. The therapist can obtain precise, detailed, sensory-based information about when, where, how, and how much the symptom always or usually occurs with respect to the following parameters or variables, among others: time of day, time of week, time of month, time of year; location in the world or in the body; frequency, rate, intensity, duration; the sequence of events in time (including all the events that consistently occur along with the symptom, i.e., "the pattern around it"); who is present; and mode or quality (depending on the symptom—voice volume; whether sitting, standing or lying down; type of food eaten on a binge; or what-have-you). These parameters of the symptom's occurrence concern the *sequence*—what follows what—and the *circumstances*—where, when, how often, how much, at what rate, with whom, and so on.

It is sometimes helpful to think of a complete description of the symptom as the answers to a hypothetical series of questions asked by someone with insatiable curiosity (as Erickson seemed to have): "How often does it happen? In what rooms of the house? Sitting or standing? Who else is around? How much? How often? When exactly? What happens first? What about after that? And then what happens?" And so on. One would thus be able to describe the "blow-by-blow" sequence of events/behaviors and the circumstances of the symptom's occurrence.

For example, at a certain point in a binge-eating pattern, a person may take a taste of some cake, or cookies, or bread, or ice cream, or chocolate (but never carrots, celery, cottage cheese, or hard-boiled eggs), and then go on a binge including all of the former items but none of the latter (i.e., if they eat "forbidden," "fat," or "nondiet" foods they typically or always binge, and they never binge on "good," "nonfattening" foods). This is followed by self-induced vomiting in the toilet, or in the sink, or in the bath (but never in the garbage can, or in a bucket, or on the carpet). And in terms of the circumstances surrounding this part of the sequence, the initial taste may be taken standing up or walking around (but never sitting or lying down), the binge-eating may take place in the kitchen, or in the dining room (but never in the bedroom or in the backyard), in the middle of the night or in mid-afternoon (but never first thing in the morning or just before bed), always alone (and never with other people around), and usually while doing nothing else in particular or sometimes while watching TV (but never while talking on the telephone or feeding the cat and dog). The pattern will have a different range — with different elements — for each person, so it is not possible to come up with some fixed "catalog" of ranges or elements or of interventions. For example, many binge-eaters binge only when alone, but some binge with others around occasionally or frequently. One needs to find out the limits of the class of things that would serve equally well to maintain the pattern as still being this particular person's binge pattern. There are many variations on the theme such that the theme remains the same theme. What one wants to introduce are variations outside those class limits that therefore define this as a new pattern. And in a new and unfamiliar pattern, anything might happen.

Modalities of Pattern Intervention

> Therapy is often a matter of tipping the first domino. (Erickson, in Rossi, 1980, Vol. 4, p. 454)

> When you have a patient with some senseless phobia, sympathize with it, and somehow or other, get them to violate that phobia. (Erickson, in Zeig, 1980, p. 253)

The discussion thus far has led to this: A sensory-based description of any invariant aspect of the sequence or circumstances of the "symptom" provides a recipe for where to intervene. "If it's invariant, vary it." In this section, there will be a brief discussion of how Erickson usually intervened in the sequence and circumstances of the symptom ("the pattern"), surveying some of the modalities of pattern intervention. The modalities to be discussed are these (using "symptom" as shorthand for the undesired experience/behavior which occurs as part of a larger pattern, the "symptom-pattern"):

1) Changing the frequency/rate of the symptom/symptom-pattern
2) Changing the duration of the symptom/symptom-pattern
3) Changing the time (of day/week/month/year) of the symptom/symptom-pattern
4) Changing the location (in the body or in the world) of the symptom/symptom-pattern
5) Changing the intensity of the symptom/symptom-pattern
6) Changing some other quality or circumstance of the symptom
7) Changing the sequence (order) of events around the symptom
8) Creating a short-circuit in the sequence (i.e., a jump from the beginning of the sequence to the end)
9) Interrupting or otherwise preventing all or part of the sequence from occurring ("derailing")
10) Adding or subtracting (at least) one element to or from the sequence
11) Breaking up any previously whole element into smaller elements
12) Having the symptom performed without the symptom-pattern
13) Having the symptom-pattern performed minus the symptom
14) Reversing the pattern

15) Linking the occurrence of the symptom-pattern to another pattern—usually an undesired experience, an avoided activity, or a desirable but difficult-to-attain goal ("symptom-contingent task")

Case examples using pattern intervention

That little hole in the dike [doesn't seem like it will] flood the land, except that it will, because once you break through an altered pattern of behavior in some way, the cracks keep traveling. (Erickson, in Haley, 1985, Vol. 1, p. 102)

Following are some cases illustrating the use of pattern intervention. Each example is followed by a notation that refers the reader back to the list of the 15 modalities for the primary type of intervention used.

In one of Erickson's cases, a 17-year-old retarded boy, recently placed in a school away from home, developed a symptom in which he rapidly waved his right arm out in front of him at a rate of 135 times per minute. (Erickson had the rate counted.) Erickson got the boy to increase the rate to 145 times per minute. Over a period of time, the rate was decreased, under Erickson's supervision, to 135 again, increased to 145, then decreased and increased by alternating an increase of five times per minute and a decrease of ten times per minute until the movement was eliminated (Rossi, 1980, Vol. 4, pp. 158–160). [Frequency/Rate, #1]

A patient of Erickson's who had delusional out-of-body trips learned to take her trips in a small amount of clock time, e.g., enjoying a three-month hallucinatory trip to her castle at the bottom of the ocean in three minutes. This, of course, resulted in her missing less time from work and seeming more "normal" to others (Rossi, 1980, Vol. 4, pp. 70–74). [Duration, #2]

A woman who suffered from asthma only during certain seasons of the year was surprised when Erickson was able to induce it during her "off season" in his office by mentioning letters she received from her father (Rossi, 1980, Vol. 4, p. 91). [Time of day/month/year, #3]

A woman with compulsive swearing (Tourette's syndrome) swore loudly only while driving alone in her car with the radio on loudly (Rossi, 1980, Vol. 4, pp. 124–130). [Location in the world, #4]

A six-year-old thumb-sucker who only sucked his left thumb was seen by Erickson. The boy was told that he was being unfair to his other digits, not giving them equal time. He was told to suck his right thumb, and eventually, each of his other fingers. Erickson remarked that as soon as the boy divided his thumb-sucking between his left and right thumb, he had in effect reduced his habit by 50 percent (Rossi, Ryan, & Sharp, 1983, p. 117). [Location in the body, #4]

The woman who had Tourette's syndrome of involuntary violent swearing and gesticulating was told to practice swearing under her breath, so that only she could hear it, and to practice making the gestures more everyday, unnoticeable movements (Rossi, 1980, Vol. 4, pp. 124–130). [Intensity, #5]

A man came to Erickson and complained that he could only urinate through a wooden or iron pipe eight to ten inches long. Erickson had the man switch to a somewhat longer bamboo pipe, and after using it for a while to begin shortening it to ten inches by degrees. He then had the man shorten it further gradually until the pipe was no longer needed (Haley, 1985, Vol. 1, pp. 153–154). [Quality of circumstances, #6]

A couple sought therapy from Erickson for marital difficulties. They ran a small restaurant together and constantly quarreled about the best way to run it. The wife insisted that the husband should be in charge, as she would rather stay home, but she feared that without her supervision he would ruin the business. So she continued to work alongside her husband and they continued to quarrel. Erickson gave them this assignment: Each morning, the husband was to go to the restaurant half an hour before his wife. When the wife arrived, the husband had already successfully fulfilled many of her "irreplaceable" functions. She started coming in even later each morning and leaving before closing, until she finally rarely showed up at the restaurant. The bickering ceased (Haley, 1973, pp. 225–226). [Sequence, #7]

A young man with a fear of traveling saw Erickson. He could drive only to the city limits. If he drove past the limits, he would vomit, then pass out. Erickson suggested that he drive to the edge of town at three in the morning, wearing his best clothes. When the young man reached the city limits, he was to stop the car and run to the shallow ditch by the side of the road. There he was to lie down until the nausea and fainting passed. Then he was to get up, drive to the next telephone pole and repeat the procedure. The man complied, but in doing the task he got so angry at Erickson and the foolishness of the procedure that he decided to just get into his car and begin to enjoy driving. Thirteen years later he was still symptom-free (Haley, 1973, pp. 69–70; Rossi, 1980, Vol. 4, pp. 134–138). [Short-circuiting, #8]

Erickson supervised a case of Zeig's (1985, p. 74) in which a dermatitis patient scratched himself while asleep, which disrupted the patient's and his wife's sleep. Erickson advised Zeig to tell the man to wrap each of his fingers with tape before going to sleep. Zeig protested that it was a long-stand-

*ing problem. Erickson replied, "Tell him to get a lot of tape."
The intervention was successful. [Derailing, #9]*

*Erickson had a woman who suffered from auditory hal-
lucinations write out everything the voices told her (Zeig,
1985, p. 70). [Adding a new element, #10]*

*A good example of breaking up a symptom was illustrated
earlier in the chapter in the case of the retired policeman who
was overweight and smoked, ate and drank too much. Erickson broke the smoking, eating, and drinking patterns into
smaller pieces. This seemed to be enough to change the patterns. [Breaking into smaller elements, #11]*

*In what surely must be one of Erickson's most bizarre cases,
he treated a couple who were both bedwetters. Through a set
of amazing circumstances, neither had been aware that the
other was a bedwetter, despite having been married for almost
a year. They were both very inhibited, religious people. They
had each been embarrassed to confess their bedwetting before
the marriage, so they faced their wedding night with some
trepidation. They had sex and fell asleep. When they awoke
the next morning to find the wet bed, each assumed the other
was being polite and understanding, as neither mentioned the
wet bed. The bedroom became associated with embarrass-
ment and inhibition, however, and they never again had sex.
A chance remark by one of them, that it would be nice if they
had a little baby on whom to blame their spot on the bed, led
them to the realization that they both wet the bed. They
resolved to get professional help and were referred by friends
to Erickson. Erickson got them to give their word that they
would do anything he told them to do to get over the problem.
He had them kneel on the bed before going to sleep each night
for three weeks and deliberately urinate on the sheets. This
was extreme torture for them. It took them several hours to*

accomplish this the first night and a long time on subsequent nights. After the three weeks, however, the bedwetting disappeared for good. The couple later had a child on whom they could blame the "spot on the bed" (Rossi, 1980, Vol. 4, pp. 99–102). [Symptom without the symptom-pattern, #12]

A nurse whom Erickson treated for severe headaches had a typical pattern associated with the headaches. She would get a headache after an emotional disturbance which involved her being generally quarrelsome with coworkers. Following the headache, she would show spasmodic movements, speak in a high-pitched voice, and speak in a sarcastic and unpleasant way to those around. Through hypnosis, Erickson was able to suggest that she have the emotional and behavioral concomitants of the headaches, but without the headaches (e.g., having the emotional disturbance followed by sleep rather than by a headache) (Rossi, 1980, Vol. 4, pp. 246–251). [Symptom pattern without the symptom, #13]

A woman sought Erickson's help for a weight problem. She reported that she had lost weight many times and would always reach her desired weight of 130 pounds. As she approached 130, she would start compulsively weighing herself. When she reached 130, she would rush to the kitchen and binge, eventually gaining back all the weight she had lost. Erickson told her that he had a diet that would work, but that she would not like it. She pleaded with him to give her a chance and gave her word to follow the diet no matter what it was. Erickson told her that she must first gain 20 pounds on his scale before she could reduce. She literally begged on her bended knees to be released from her promise. Each pound she gained, the more desperate she became. When she finally reached 200, Erickson helped her reduce to 130. She vowed that she would never gain again after the agony of that 20 pounds. Erickson commented that he had reversed her

usual pattern of reduce, then gain (Rosen, 1982, pp. 123–125).
[Reversing the pattern, #14]

(The next section will take up the subject of symptom
contingent tasks in more detail, with several case examples,
so no symptom contingent cases have been included in this
section.)

Symptom-contingent tasks

> The idea is to make a laborious task out of whatever the
> habit is — you turn a vicious habit into an awful inconven-
> ience which the patient is very willing to give up. (Erickson,
> in Rossi, Ryan, & Sharp, 1983, p. 264)

In *Strategies of Psychotherapy* (Haley, 1963) and *Ordeal
Therapy* (Haley, 1984), Jay Haley wrote about a class of interventions in Erickson's work which he called "benevolent ordeals." Haley (1963, p. 55) writes, "The basic rule of brief
psychotherapy would seem to be to encourage the symptom
in such a way that the patient cannot continue to utilize it.
One of the quickest methods is to persuade the patient to
punish himself when he suffers from the symptom, thereby
encouraging him to give up the symptom." Benevolent ordeals
can be considered a type of pattern intervention (#15 in the
list). This section specifies some unrecognized aspects of this
class of interventions, gives a structure to the interventions,
and renames the class "symptom-contingent tasks."

Symptom-contingent tasks are behavioral homework assignments given by the therapist. When the symptom occurs, the
patient is to perform the assignment. A case from my clinical
practice serves to illustrate the use of this technique.

*A professional woman sought treatment to stop compulsive
bingeing on food. Relevant information gathered indicated*

that the woman's husband liked to debate almost nightly. He enjoyed a good argument. My client, however, disliked this style of interaction and tried to ignore his attempts to start a debate. At times she would be provoked and at other times she was able to resist joining the argument. She often binged after these debates. She had asked him to stop. He hadn't and she had resignedly decided that this was the way he was and there was nothing she could do about it. She had, moreover, binged before she was married to him.

It was also discovered that, while assertive in other areas, she was situationally non-assertive in the marriage. Although she wanted to spend more time alone and with friends, she found herself acquiescing to her husband's demand that she spend all her leisure time with him. She did not do much housework, however, although her husband expected her to and complained when she did not. She reported that she hated housework.

Her homework assignment was to: (1) Time the debates and spend the same amount of time the next night alone or with friends; and (2) each time she binged, to do an hour's worth of housework. Her reply to this second aspect of the assignment was, "An hour's worth of housework! I'll never binge!" She agreed to the assignment. She never binged again and became more assertive in the marriage. She reported amazement that it had been so easy and said that, any time she considered bingeing, she didn't do it because she knew she would then have to keep her promise to do an hour's worth of housework.

With this general understanding of symptom-contingent tasks, let us look at the method of constructing these tasks for patients. The first step in formulating this type of intervention is to gather information from the person about the presenting complaint and surrounding patterns or context. Then the therapist determines whether to concentrate more on intervening with just the individual, with the interpersonal aspects, or with both. The example above included both interpersonal and personal interventions.

The binge-housework assignment dealt mainly with the individual client. Both the task and the symptom were under her influence, although this assignment might have had an effect on the interpersonal aspects of the symptom context. The assignment related to debates and independent time clearly dealt with a more interpersonal aspect. She had little direct control over the debates.

The next step is to ask about some other desired goal or difficulty, personal or interpersonal. Usually, in individually focused situations, this can best be elicited by asking, "Is there anything you think you should do, but procrastinate about or don't do, like housework, correspondence, cleaning the front closet, etc.?" In interpersonally focused situations, the question might be, "Is there anything that you like to do that the other person doesn't like for you to do (and that isn't illegal or immoral)?"

The final step is to link some significant (by the patient's definition) amount of time or effort at this neglected or avoided behavior with the occurrence of the symptom or unwanted behavior. Then, of course, the therapist must obtain the patient's agreement.

It may be that sometimes the person doesn't even have to do the assignment for it to have the therapeutic effect (as the case example above illustrates). Haley has focused on the "ordeal" aspect of the directive, but Erickson, with his emphasis on personal and social utility, often linked the symptom to tasks that would lead to some desirable personal or social goal.

> You see to it that the patient discovers that there are a number of other things that he would rather be doing, and you make it awfully easy for him to discontinue the particular habit. (Erickson, in Rossi, Ryan, & Sharp, 1982, p. 265)

The following case examples, from Erickson's clinical practice as well as my own, illustrate the use of this class of intervention.

A 29-year-old man always wet his bed between midnight and 1 a.m. Erickson instructed him to get an alarm clock and set it for midnight or for half past twelve or for one o'clock. When the alarm rang, he was to get up and walk 40 blocks, regardless of whether the bed was wet or dry. He was to do this for the next three weeks. Erickson had discovered prior to the assignment that the man hated to walk. After the three weeks, he could have a week's vacation, but the next time after that when he found a wet bed he was to serve another three weeks' sentence of walking 40 blocks in the middle of the night (Rossi, Ryan, & Sharp, 1983, pp. 264–265).

Erickson told a man who wanted to stop smoking that he was to put an equivalent value in coins in a jar every time he lit up a cigarette (Gordon & Meyers-Anderson, 1981, p. 21).

A lawyer sought the author's help, asking for hypnosis to help stop smoking. He was told that hypnosis would be used only on the condition that he agree to an assignment. The lawyer indicated that he had quite a bit of paperwork at home and at the office. He agreed that if he smoked after the appointment, he would do 15 minutes of neglected paperwork before he smoked another cigarette.

A couple sought therapy from me. The husband was, they both agreed, a "workaholic." He constantly promised he would be on time, but he was consistently late from work. The wife would talk to him about it, and he would promise anew and arrive home on time for a while, but gradually he would drift back into his late pattern. She was considering divorce. He didn't like her to go out with her girlfriends and didn't par-

*ticularly like to visit either his or her parents, which she liked
to do on the weekend. The assignment to which they agreed
was that, whenever he wasn't home by 8 p.m., she was to keep
track of how many minutes he was late. She could then spend
an equivalent amount of time either going out with girlfriends
and/or having them both spend time visiting their parents on
Sunday.*

*A woman in her thirties reported that she had sucked her
thumb and scratched her nipple and belly button until they
scabbed. She requested therapy from Erickson, but he told
her he wasn't going to give her therapy, he was just going to
cure her in 30 seconds. All she had to do was to agree to come
in to Erickson's office and scratch her nipple in front of him
the next time she had the urge to do it (Haley, 1985, Vol. 1,
p. 15).*

*An older gentleman whose wife had died had developed
a severe case of insomnia. He was getting only two hours of
sleep per night on average, although he spent 14 or 15 hours
in bed tossing and turning most of the time. Erickson discovered that the man hated to wax the wooden floors in his
house, as he had to wax them by hand and he hated the smell
of the floor wax. He got the man to agree to wax the floors
all night when he couldn't sleep. The man was able to overcome the insomnia after just two nights of floor waxing (Haley,
1985, Vol. 1, pp. 54–55).*

There are many previously unrecognized or underempha-
sized aspects of symptom-contingent interventions in Erickson's work. While this approach could be viewed as a variation
on the behavioral approach of contingency management, several of these aspects suggest something beyond punishment
as an explanation for its efficacy.

One unrecognized aspect of symptom-contingent tasks is

that they can actually accomplish two goals at once. Patients often both make progress towards the elimination of the symptom and complete avoided tasks. A case of Erickson's illustrates:

> *I remember one woman who said, "I want you to make it hard for me to smoke." I said, "I can suggest ways . . . it's up to you to keep it hard." She said, "And I know what will be hard. I'm overweight. Have me keep my cigarettes in the basement, and my matches in the attic, and I can only have one cigarette at a time, and I have to go down to the basement to get it, and I have to go up into the attic to light it. That amount of exercise will reduce my weight." And she got so interested in weight loss she quit smoking. She had a new goal, so she accomplished two things (Erickson, in Gordon & Meyers-Anderson, 1981, pp. 21-22)*

Another example of Erickson's work suggests a different unrecognized aspect.

> *A 12-year-old boy was in an intense struggle with his mother over his continued wetting of the bed. Erickson gave mother the assignment of waking up at 4 or 5 a.m. every night to check whether her son's bed was wet or dry. If it was dry, she was to go back to bed without waking the boy. If it was wet, she was to get the boy up and have him practice his handwriting (which was very poor) until 7 a.m. Not only was the symptom resolved, but the boy's friendships, relationship with his parents, and grades at school improved (Haley, 1973, pp. 206-208).*

One aspect of this intervention that is not readily apparent is that Erickson assigned a task which was in some ways parallel to the desired outcome: learning muscle control. Mother and son had been struggling over the son's developing muscle control while asleep; Erickson reoriented their struggle

to something that the boy could deliberately practice to gain
muscle control—handwriting. Both mother and son could see
his steady improvement in this area, and a similar increase in
muscle control became evident in his bedwetting. This topic
will be discussed in more detail in Chapter 4 on parallel communication. While there are other aspects of this case, it is
enough here to suggest that symptom-contingent tasks can
have further implications and effects than might be obvious
at first glance.

The cases discussed here have shown a major aspect of
Erickson's nonhypnotic (sometimes called "strategic") work.
He was very focused on introducing change directly into the
rigid symptom pattern. Of course, this approach was sometimes seen in his hypnotic work, when, for example, he would
move a headache to a different location or alter the sensation
of the headache from sharp to dull. In fact, a case could be
made for pattern intervention as the primary principle that
connects all of Erickson's work, but here it is used in a more
limited, technical sense.

ESTABLISHING NEW PATTERNS

Once Erickson, after unsuccessfully attempting to establish
rapport with a rather disturbed patient, took off his coat and
put it on backwards and inside out. He then took off the
patient's coat and put it on the patient backwards and inside
out. Establishing this new pattern was the beginning of a
successful relationship (Rosen, 1982, pp. 198–199).

The most extensive examples of establishing new patterns
from Erickson's work involve "Harold," the farm laborer with
whom Erickson worked for several years and saw from an
unkempt, insecure illiterate farmhand to a well-groomed, so-
phisticated college graduate (Haley, 1973, pp. 120–148), and
the woman in the case called "The February Man," for whom
Erickson provided new childhood memories via hypnosis.

This woman had little experience with nurturing parents and wanted to be a good parent for the child she was expecting (Erickson & Rossi, 1979, pp. 461–477). These cases are too lengthy to detail here, but in both cases Erickson established new patterns in the behavioral and experiential lives of the patients.

A case which is more amenable to summary here is one in which a husband and wife sought marital therapy with Erickson. The wife was dissatisfied with the husband's pattern of asking her to go out to eat and then deciding which restaurant they would go to (one of five favorites of his) and what she would eat, despite her objections. He was always very pleasant about it and couched it all in a way that seemed to express concern (e.g., "You wouldn't like that. Why don't you order this?"). The husband, a very meticulous man, was abashed by his wife's complaint and denied it. Erickson proceeded to get a map and dictate a very elaborate set of driving instructions that would take the couple on a roundabout route to a new restaurant. When they arrived there, the wife (acting on Erickson's private instructions) switched menus with her husband before they had a chance to look at them. As soon as both had had a chance to make their food choices, she switched menus again. She ordered what she wanted and expressed her gratitude to her husband at the end of the night. He had never experienced her gratitude before, as she had always been resentful. He suggested they follow a similar procedure the next time they went out. So they took a roundabout route of his choosing and she chose the restaurant — the first good one after the route ended. Erickson also discovered that the wife had been upset because, when the husband bought her flowers, they were never for her, but always as a centerpiece for the table, very functional and very ornate. Erickson suggested that the husband get a florist to make up a random selection of mismatched flowers and wrap them in an out-of-town news-

paper. She was delighted. Erickson also suggested that, instead of meeting the wife's expectations for their next anniversary (a big, elaborate dinner with friends at a private dining room), the man arrange a surprise camping trip for them. He did and again she was delightfully surprised. These changes resulted in the establishment of new patterns for the couple, along the lines that Erickson had suggested (but individualized by them) (Haley, 1985, Vol. 2, pp. 33-42).

Some typical techniques that Erickson used to establish new patterns are detailed below.

The Yes Set

A technique commonly used by Erickson was to establish a habit or set of agreement from patients or audiences to make them more receptive to ideas and cooperation. He called this a "yes set." For example, he might, during an interview, ask a series of questions which he knew were likely to elicit an affirmative response, such as, "You have sought my help for a problem, right?" and "I am a psychiatrist, correct?" After several questions like this, he would ask a question that would not have such an obvious answer, but was a leading one with which Erickson wanted the person to agree, such as, "And you would like to go into a trance, would you not?" (Erickson, Rossi, & Rossi, 1976, pp. 58-59).

The Reverse Set

Here is an example of this technique, taken from Erickson's hypnotic induction with a woman named Ruth:

Erickson: "And now I want you to shake your head No. [Erickson models head shaking.] Your name isn't Ruth, is it? [Erickson shakes No; Ruth shakes No.] And you aren't a woman, are you? [Ruth shakes her head No.] And you aren't sitting down, are you? [Ruth shakes her head No.] And you aren't in trance, are you? [Ruth shakes her head No.]" (Erickson & Rossi, 1981, pp. 166–167)

Erickson used this repatterning maneuver at times in hypnotic inductions and treatment. The essence of the technique was to get subjects or patients to shake their head (no) when the answer they wanted to give was "yes" and to nod their head (yes) when their answer was "no" (Erickson & Rossi, 1981, pp. 163–168). This usually had several effects. The first and foremost was confusion. It takes some thinking to reverse one's lifelong habitual response. The more confusing the questions or the faster they were offered, the more likely the subject would become very confused. This was one of Erickson's goals in inducing a trance: to confuse and distract the subject's conscious vigilance and self-imposed limitations so that new experiences could emerge.

Another effect was to have the person break up an old pattern and establish a new one, which, as we have seen, was compatible with Erickson's goals in therapy. It could be seen as an indirect or parallel message to the person with regard to the symptom: If one habitual pattern can change, then another (the symptom pattern) can as well.

Thirdly, this technique established a split or a disconnection between the subject's thinking and action. This can also be viewed as a parallel message: Your thinking does not have to determine your behavior in this area or in the symptom area.

The No Set

A heckler in the audience forced Erickson to stop his lecture with his frequent and loud comments. Erickson challenged the man and told him " . . . that he had to remain silent; that he could not speak again; that he did not dare to stand up;

that he could not again charge fraud; . . . " — all things the man refused to do. Erickson then told the man that he was afraid to come up to the stage, that he was afraid to look at the demonstration subjects, that he did not dare to remain silent, that he did not dare to listen to Erickson, that he did not dare to walk to one of the demonstration chairs, that he would not sit down, that he would put his hands behind his head rather than resting them on his thighs, etc. The heckler (or rather the former heckler, since Erickson had dared him to silence) was soon resisting all of Erickson's predictions and dares, thereby cooperating completely with a trance induction. He subsequently developed a deep trance (Rossi, 1980, Vol. 1, pp. 192-193). Erickson established a "no set," in which the client disputed everything he said. Then Erickson merely ordered the man to do the opposite of what he (Erickson) wanted.

SUMMARY AND OVERVIEW
OF PATTERN INTERVENTION

It must be remembered that patterns are not "things." Yet they are the next best thing to "things." They are descriptive abstractions. When observing some actions, an observer can abstract *patterns* of action. This does not involve theorizing or explaining the existence of these facts, speculating about what function they serve, or other forms of "psychologizing." It is more like classifying organisms into species or objects into a set.

Some therapists might object to dealing only with the behavioral aspects of the symptoms. "What about the feelings?" they might inquire. William James spoke to this concern succinctly when he wrote, "Action seems to follow feeling, but really action and feeling go together; and by regulating the action, which is under the more direct control of the will, we can use it to indirectly regulate the feeling, which is not."

And what about the underlying problem? Aren't pattern

interventions just dealing with the surface manifestations? Erickson used the analogy of a boiling pot on a stove to meet this objection. Isn't it easier, he said, to move the pot around by the handle than by grasping the hot pot directly? Symptoms are like the handle (Haley, 1982, p. 19).

Erickson used another analogy when he discussed pattern intervention. He said it was a lot of effort to dam up a flowing river, but it took a lot less effort to channel that river in another direction. Pattern intervention was his method of "channeling" the patient's behavior and experience. Sometimes this channeling was done to work towards other goals in therapy and sometimes the goal was simply to change unworkable patterns and to eliminate the symptom.

3. *Splitting and Linking*

> There are two types of people in the world: those who
> divide people into two parts and those who don't.
>
> —John Barth

Erickson used, as much as possible, existing skills, behaviors, and patterns of human experience to effect changes. One of the patterns he often mentioned was that of "mental mechanisms." These mental mechanisms include the complementary patterns of splitting and linking. These might even be considered as one pattern, since they rarely occur in isolation from one another.

Erickson's work makes use of the natural propensity of people to make distinctions (splitting) and associations (linking). These tendencies are used to break up previous associations and to make new distinctions and new associations, which will facilitate the realization of therapeutic goals.

SPLITTING

> . . . a universe comes into being when a space is severed or
> taken apart. . . . By tracing the way we represent such a
> severance, we can begin . . . to see how the familiar laws of
> our own experience follow inexorably from the original act
> of severance. (Brown, 1972, p. v)

People tend to conceptually split their world up into pieces. We talk of A.D. and B.C. (and indeed, of hours and days), al-

54

though there is no inherent division in time. Studies of social behavior show that we create divisions in space to mark territory. We split our planet into separate countries. We use rites of passage to separate developmental and social stages. We break large tasks into smaller pieces in order to make them more manageable. It is a natural thing for people to make divisions in their behavior and in their experience. We make distinctions to make sense of the world and to organize our perceptions, behavior, and experience.

Erickson used this natural tendency to induce trances and to provide therapeutic interventions. He created a context that was structured and divided in very particular ways to help people obtain therapeutic results. At times he would give a task assignment that would have the result of breaking up the previous symptom-supporting context or pattern (see Chapter 2). At other times he would structure both his verbal and nonverbal communications to help people dissociate one part of their experience from another. He might talk about an "unconscious mind" and a "conscious mind," using each of those terms with different associated voice dynamics and body positions. Or he might ask people in trance to wake up just as a mind, but to let their bodies stay in trance. In various ways, both in hypnotic and nonhypnotic settings, he created a context for breaking up previously whole units into (at least) two parts or cleaving previously associated elements in experience or behavior.

Patients often make distinctions, punctuations, or splits in the "problem" arena that are not useful, i.e., these particular splits bring about an unwanted experience or result. For example, the split between mind and body can be seen to have some unfortunate consequences for those with "psychosomatic" problems. Below are examples from Erickson's work in which he skillfully uses the operation of splitting to make more useful distinctions and punctuations with his patients. Explanatory comments are enclosed in brackets.

A patient with neuralgia was told " . . . that the first bite of
the filet mignon would be painful but that the rest of it would
be so very good . . . " (Rossi, 1980, Vol. 1, p. 330). [Split = first
bite/all subsequent bites]

Erickson described a situation in which a patient was told
to sit in a certain chair to go into trance, and " . . . thereafter
merely sitting in that chair induced a trance. When the therapist did not wish him to develop a trance, he was simply asked
to sit in another chair . . . " (Rossi, 1980, Vol. 1, p. 310). [Split
= this chair/that chair]

A patient couldn't develop the oral anesthesia he desired
for dental work and in fact became orally hypersensitive,
although he could readily develop hypnotic anesthesia in all
other parts of his body. Erickson induced a trance and instructed the patient to develop hypersensitivity in one of his
hands. The patient achieved the requested hand hypersensitivity and concomitantly developed the desired oral anesthesia
(Rossi, 1980, Vol. 1, p. 169). [Split = hand/rest of body; hyper-
esthesia/anesthesia]

A dentist's wife couldn't go into trance because every time
an induction was initiated she became "scared stiff," couldn't
move, and then started crying. Erickson explained to her
that it was enough to be stiff without the necessity of crying
right away. Then he had her go into a trance by making her
eyelids stiff so that she couldn't move them after her eyes
were closed. Then he instructed her to get scared silly and
then cry, but not just yet . . . " (Rossi, 1980, Vol. 1, p. 169).
[Split = scared/stiff/crying]

A patient of Erickson's after being hypnotized, claimed that
the hypnosis had not really been effective, because he re-
embered everything that Erickson had said. Erickson replied

that of course *the patient could remember everything* here. *He was* here *in the office, it all occurred* here *and* here *he could remember everything. The patient developed amnesia for the trance experience everywhere but inside Erickson's office (Rossi, 1980, Vol. 1, p. 191). [Split = memory in the office/memory outside the office]*

Erickson told a woman who was fearful of consummating her marriage that the consummation should occur within the next ten days, but that he (Erickson) preferred Friday as the day. He kept reiterating his choice of days. "A dilemma she could not recognize of two alternatives was created for her— the day of her choice or of the writer's preference . . . " (Rossi, 1980, Vol. 4, p. 170). [Split = Friday/all other days of the week]

" . . . Then you point out to a patient that it's perfectly possible to remember the intellectual facts of something but not the emotional content . . . " (Erickson, 1964). [Split = intellect/emotion]

Erickson, in his treatment of a six-year-old boy who sucked his thumb and chewed his fingernails excessively, told the boy that he should go ahead and suck his thumb and chew his nails all he wanted. Erickson said that "a little six-year-old" needs to do these things. Of course, a "seven-year-old big kid" will be "too big and too old" to do these things. Before his seventh birthday, which was two months later, the boy stopped sucking his thumb and chewing his nails (Zeig, 1980, pp. 112–113). [Split = six-year-old little boy/seven-year-old big boy]

These examples illustrate the technique of splitting in its myriad forms in therapeutic work. If carefully examined, they can also be seen to contain examples of the complementary process of linking, as will be discussed later.

Erickson also used the operation of splitting in his nonverbal communication. He used certain body positions, voice tones, voice volumes, and voice locations (cf. Bandler and Grinder's (1975) discussions of *analogical marking* and Erickson's discussions of the *interspersal technique*). This use of splitting will be discussed in more detail in Chapter 9.

One indication for the use of splitting is when elements of a system (whether intra- or inter-personal) are struggling with each other with equal force. The situation can perhaps be likened to traffic jams or gridlock, in which the cars from both directions are blocking intersections. If some traffic could be diverted, it would free up the rest of the traffic and the traffic jam would clear on its own.

An example is Erickson's approach to a woman who said she wanted to go into a trance, but, despite having seen three previous hypnotists, hadn't been able to do so. Erickson reports that "with two markedly differing inflections and tempo the following was said to her as a two-part statement, 'I CAN'T HYPNOTIZE YOU, justyourarm." The trance induction was successful (Rossi, 1980, Vol. 1, pp. 288–290).

Different techniques for accomplishing this therapeutic splitting are discussed below.

Illusion of Alternatives

The technique of illusion of alternatives (sometimes called "double bind" by Erickson) consists of giving the patient at least two options. Whichever option is chosen will lead to the desired result. Most parents know this technique. "Would you like to have a story read to you or watch 15 more minutes of television before you go to bed?" Erickson used it in both hypnotic contexts and nonhypnotic therapy. "Do you think that eliminating this problem in two weeks or three weeks is more realistic?" "Would you like to go into trance now or later in the session?"

Apposition of Opposites; Oxymoron

These are two similar techniques of splitting. The first, apposition of opposites, is the use of two polar concepts or experiences in the same context or sentence (Erickson, Rossi, & Rossi, 1976, pp. 201–202). "You can *remember* to *forget* what is unimportant." "As one hand *lifts*, the other can *lower*." "It's interesting how you can be *comfortable* even about things which are *uncomfortable*."

Oxymoron (from the Greek *oxys* [sharp] + *moros* [dull, foolish]) is the second technique. Here the opposites are included in one phrase, as in "same difference," "burning cold," and "sweet sorrow." In one of Erickson's cases, a woman who was promiscuous but very afraid of men and sex was advised by Erickson that she could take a "vicious pleasure" in her ability to turn a man's hard, threatening penis into a limp, helpless object (Rosen, 1982, pp. 36–37).

Dissociation

Dissociation is a widely recognized psychological and hypnotic phenomenon. People can separate psychological states (such as "parent," "adult," and "child" in transactional analysis or the simple distinctions of "conscious" and "unconscious" or "awake" and "asleep"), emotions from thinking, behavior from feeling, etc. In some therapeutic problems, patients have used dissociation in a harmful way, but Erickson used the same "mental mechanism" to benefit patients in hypnosis and therapy.

The hypnotic technique of having subjects view their past traumatic incidents as if they were on a movie screen while their body remains relaxed and comfortable is an example of dissociation.

Splitting in Time

With a mother, father and daughter who were always arguing, Erickson arranged that they should argue in his office. Each would have 20 minutes to have his or her say. Using the principle of "age before beauty and ladies first," mother went first, daughter went second, and father went last (Haley, 1985, Vol. 3, pp. 49–50).

Splitting Roles

To a mother who was having difficulty letting her last son move away from home, Erickson said that she was making the transition from good mother of the past to potential grandmother of the future (Haley, 1985, Vol. 3, p. 24).

Body/Voice Splitting and Interspersal

Erickson investigated the effect of different voice locations and tones on hypnotic phenomena. He used these different body positions and tones to distinguish between different messages. He might sway his body back and forth, thereby suggesting a boat voyage for people who had heard similar voice changes while conversing on a previous voyage (Rossi, 1980, Vol. 2, pp. 121–141). He might turn his head to the right to give one set of messages, say for the unconscious, and to the left to give another set of messages, for the conscious mind. This was his main method for delivering interspersed suggestions in therapy. "Interspersal" is the name of a technique in which the therapist nonverbally emphasizes certain phrases to give subliminal suggestions to the patient. Erickson's best-known case of this (mentioned earlier) involved "Joe," the florist, who was suffering from severe pain while dying of cancer (Rossi, 1980, Vol. 4, pp. 262–278). With Joe, Erickson launched into a long, specious discussion of tomato plants, which included interspersed suggestions (distinguished by a different voice volume, tone and location) like "sense of comfort," "feel very good, feel very comfortable," "growing comfortably," etc. Joe was able to go into trance and achieve pain control with these suggestions.

Reject One (or the Worst) Alternative

An inhibited young woman in treatment with Erickson was told that at the next appointment she was to bring the "shortest pair of short shorts imaginable" and show them to him. When she did, he told her that at the next appointment she had a choice — she could bring them with her and put them on in front of him or she could come to the session dressed in the shorts. Part of his treatment with her involved desensitizing her to the subject of sex. When he tried to talk with her about sex, she would develop deafness. He told her that she would now listen to him as he discussed sex or he would have her take off the shorts and put them on again in his presence. She listened (Haley, 1985, Vol. 2, p. 127).

LINKING

We used to think that if we knew one, we knew two, because one and one are two. We are finding that we must learn a great deal more about *"and"* (Sir Arthur Stanley Eddington).

Linking is the joining together of two (or more) elements that previously had no such association. Following are examples from Erickson's work.

*"He was told to close his eyes and repeat his story from
beginning to end, to do this slowly, carefully . . . and as he did
so, the mere sound of his own voice would serve to induce
in him a satisfactory trance . . . " (Rossi, 1980, Vol. 1, p. 208).
[Link = the sound of the man's voice reciting his story slowly
will induce trance]*

*" . . . noting that the author was writing down each of his
statements, the patient slowed his speech to accommodate
the author's writing speed . . . " (Rossi, 1980, Vol. 1, p. 311).
[link = Erickson's note-taking linked with the patient's rate
of speech]*

*" . . . just look at that paperweight . . . by looking at it, you
will hold your eyes still and that will hold your head still and
that will hold your ears still . . . " (Rossi, 1980, Vol. 1, p. 302).
[links = looking at paperweight will cause eyes to hold still;
holding eyes still will hold head and ears still]*

*"And then I said, 'Now of course, whenever I count to
twenty, you can go into a hypnotic trance.' . . . Then I looked
at them significantly and said, 'I had four boys and four girls —
that makes eight. They really come cheaper by the dozen, you
know.' With that they both went into a trance. Eight and
twelve is twenty" (Rossi, 1980, Vol. 1, p. 297). [link = counting
to twenty will induce a trance]*

*" . . . casual remarks were made about inhaling and exhaling,
these words timed to fit in with her actual breathing. Others
were made about the ease with which she could almost automatically lift her cigarette to her mouth and then lower her
hand to the arm of the chair. These remarks were also timed
to coincide with her actual behavior. Soon the words 'inhale',
'exhale,' 'lift,' and 'lower' acquired a conditioning value of
which she was unaware because of the seemingly conversa-*

tional character of the suggestions. Similarly, casual sugges-
tions were offered in which the words 'sleep,' 'sleepy,' and
'sleeping' were timed to her eyelid behavior . . . " (Rossi, 1980,
Vol. 1, p. 152). [links = words "inhale" and "exhale" linked with
behavior of inhaling and exhaling; eyelids closing linked to
words "sleep," "sleepy," and "sleeping"]

From these and other hypnotic experiments, Erickson
learned how readily people respond to these artificially at-
tributed linkages, which he readily used to facilitate the induction of trance and the attainment of therapeutic goals.
Several categories of linking are discussed below.

Symptom Transformation

Symptom transformation is a technique developed by Erickson for taking the underlying emotion or energy of a problem
and linking it to a different object. With obsessive patients,
Erickson would often get them to obsess in some way that
would lead to symptom resolution. For example, he would
arrange for them to become obsessed about what day their
symptoms would disappear and what they would do after their
symptom disappeared with all the energy and time that used
to go into the symptom.

Erickson reported that he often told premature ejaculators
that they had probably never been told the eventual outcome
of premature ejaculation. Sooner or later they will experience
the frustration of not being able to ejaculate. "They're using
the same mechanisms, a state of expectancy, of defeat, in
relationship to the ejaculation" (Erickson, 1960).
In another case, a man with phantom limb pain was told
that phantom limb pain can become phantom limb pleasure
(Erickson & Rossi, 1979, pp. 106–120).
Erickson suggested to a man with a stammer that a stammer

*was an expression of anger towards others. The manner in
which Erickson suggested this to the patient elicited anger.
When the man got angry at Erickson he no longer had the
symptom. After he realized this, he decided to be angry at
Erickson, as Erickson was "a nice guy to hate" (Rossi, 1980,
Vol. 4, pp. 92–93).*

Constructing New Associations

With a woman whose adult son was still living at home and
who thought that Erickson did not understand her, Erickson
constructed two new linkages. Whenever she mentioned that
Erickson did not understand her, Erickson said that since her
son was still living at home she could understand her son.
Whenever she got the feeling Erickson understood her, he
mentioned the possibility of her son's living away from home.
After some time, the woman became more amenable to the
prospect of her son's moving away (Haley, 1985, Vol. 3, pp.
31–32).

Contingent Suggestions

Erickson often used suggestions that implied a causal connection, however specious those suggestions may have been
when analyzed by a critical observer. These are suggestions
like, "If your arm lifts up to your face, then your unconscious
is working for you," and, "As you sit in that chair, you can go
all the way into trance." It might be that the intensity of some
experience or behavior is linked to another, e.g., "The more
your conscious mind is distracted, the easier it will be for your
unconscious mind to help you go into a trance."

Posthypnotic suggestion is another type of a contingent
suggestion. At some time or event in the future, after the
trance is over, the patient will behave in some particular way
or will have some experience.

Time Suggestions for Symptom Resolution

At times Erickson casually gave suggestions for a time frame for symptom resolution. He might say to a boy with enuresis that he would not expect him to have a dry bed within a week—that would be too soon. He would not expect it in two weeks, but he could not be as certain of that. He would be very surprised if the boy did not start having dry beds in two months, however. In another case, he suggested that sometime between St. Patrick's Day and April Fool's Day, a boy's symptom could be resolved.

SIMULTANEOUS
SPLITTING AND LINKING

The discerning reader may have noticed that for every split there is an implied link and vice versa. Here we will examine the joint use of the two operations in a more explicit way.

An example of the simultaneous use of splitting and linking was the treatment of a woman with a severe case of psoriasis who reluctantly sought therapy from Erickson and who very reluctantly agreed to show him the hideous scaling of her arms. Erickson told her, after examining her, "You haven't got more than a third of the psoriasis that you think you have." She reacted angrily to this obvious insult to her intelligence and to the implication that it was "all in her head." He continued, "You have a little psoriasis and a lot of emotions." She angrily wrote him a check "for his time" and terminated therapy. She called Erickson in two weeks, however, stating that she had been furious at him for the entire two weeks and that each day her psoriasis had cleared up more and more, until she now had little left (Rosen, 1982, pp. 154–155).

Here Erickson had proposed a split (psoriasis = a little psoriasis + a lot of emotions) and then arranged for her to experience a lot of emotion. The more she experienced the emotions, the less psoriasis she had.

ANCHORING THE
RESISTANCE/SYMPTOM

Erickson had many innovative means of avoiding or ameliorating resistance in therapy. One of his techniques was to allow the patient or subject to have his resistance, but to limit the expression of the resistance to a certain location or a certain time or subject, one that would not interfere with the therapeutic or hypnotic work. I label this technique "anchoring the resistance." He used a similar technique with symptoms, limiting their expression to a certain time or place. I label this "anchoring the symptom." Erickson gave a nice analogy to illustrate this principle. If a farmer with prime hunting land on his farm puts up a "No trespassing" sign, the hunters will sneak onto his land to hunt. If, however, the farmer meets with the hunters and tells them that they can hunt on a specific parcel of ground, they are much more likely to remain in that area (Haley, 1985, Vol. 3, p. 29).

Anchoring the Resistance

> In therapy your patient is going to offer you resistances of all kinds. Well, you ask them to put that resistance in a certain place. Where it's handy, where it's ready, where it's useful. He sort of keeps his eye on it right there where he can use it. And you walk around. But he did come to you for help, and you keep stepping under his guard by that shift of context. (Erickson, in Haley, 1985, Vol. 2, p. 131)

If a patient appeared to offer resistance, Erickson would channel and prescribe the resistance, but in a way that limited its effects on therapy. One way for patients to show resistance is to withhold crucial information from the therapist. A woman patient was giving Erickson her history and he noticed she had left out six years of her life. When he pointed this out to her, she told him that she was reluctant to tell him about that period. He said, "All right, think it over carefully. Now what part of that six years don't you want to tell me?" She proceeded to tell him about all the years but 1927. After she had told him those other years, she decided she might as well go ahead and tell him about 1927 (Haley, 1985, Vol. 2, pp. 131–132).

Anchoring the Symptom

Erickson treated a woman with an airplane phobia. She was put into trance and given suggestions to hallucinate being in the air. She showed all her usual "phobic" reactions. Then she was told that as soon as the plane landed (in her hallucination), all her fears and phobias would slide off her body and onto the seat beside her. She awoke free of the phobia, but thereafter would not allow anyone to sit in that chair, as her phobia was now anchored to that particular place. The simultaneous splitting and linking were accomplished by splitting the phobia from her body and linking the phobia to the chair. (Zeig, 1980, p. 66)

An 82-year-old physician dying of cancer was a patient of Erickson's. Erickson was doing hypnotic pain control with the man. The man described a "continuous, deadly, killing pain" throughout his body. Erickson discussed with the man the well-known phenomenon of "displaced" or "referred" pain, in which the original trauma occurred in one area, but was experienced as pain in another part of the body. When one has a coronary, the pain is felt in the left arm, despite the fact that the main trauma occurs to the heart. In a similar manner, he told the physician that the whole body pain was what was

*killing him, and Erickson suggested that if he had all that
"killing pain" in just his left hand, he probably wouldn't mind
it as much. The man agreed and developed a severe pain in
his left hand (he was right-handed). The pain had been split
into pieces and linked to one part of his body, his left hand.
(Rossi, Ryan, & Sharp, 1983, pp. 229–230)*

*A woman with hallucinations of nude men floating above
her head when she arrived in Erickson's office was persuaded
to leave them in Erickson's office closet. Next she developed
psychotic episodes and Erickson got her to put each one in
a manila envelope and bring them to him. This served to keep
her functioning adequately in her job and with other people.
The woman visited the office occasionally to either drop off
or look at her psychotic episode envelopes. Erickson kept them
for many years, even though the woman moved to another
city. She occasionally traveled to check on her envelopes
where her symptoms were anchored. (Rossi, 1980, Vol. 4, pp.
73–74)*

Erickson acted almost as an editor of human experience,
perception, and behavior, cutting here and splicing there.
From earlier experience with hypnosis he had discovered how
malleable human meanings are. The operations of splitting
and linking are ways of constructing more useful meanings
and outcomes for psychotherapy patients.

4. Parallel Communication

... [the healer should not tell] the naked truth. He should use images, allegories, figures, wonderous speech, or other hidden roundabout ways.

—Paracelsus (in Pachter, 1982, p. 63)

Erickson often communicated in metaphor. He talked about one topic to indirectly refer to another. He preferred an indirect, metaphorical approach that allowed people to make their own meanings (as opposed to having those meanings imposed by well-meaning therapists), thinking that therapy patients were the least likely to benefit from a direct approach. In discussing his bias against a direct approach, Erickson said, " . . . you can't let your patient — he wouldn't be your patient if he could handle it directly — know too much about it, or else he will consciously, deliberately improve upon your ideas" (Haley, 1985, Vol. 2, pp. 121–122). This deliberate improvement would, in Erickson's view, lead to more of the same problem, as the patient has probably already tried what he consciously believes will solve the problem. Erickson preferred to use parallel communication to indirectly provide therapy.

What is included under the heading of parallel communication? *Jokes* are used to humorously and indirectly make points that would have been pedantic or resistance-provoking if made directly. For example, the rather overbearing stepfather might not respond well if told directly that perhaps his views on childrearing were not the *best* or the *only* views possible. But, when told the following joke, he might be more receptive to relaxing his "expert" pose:

> I have heard about a lecturer who built up a great reputa-
> tion as an expert on child education, though he had never
> married himself. The title of his lectures was "Ten Com-
> mandments for Parents." Then he met the girl of his
> dreams, married her, and became a father. Shortly there-
> after he changed the title of his talk to "Ten Hints for
> Parents." He was blessed with a second offspring—and his
> talk was relabeled "A Few Tentative Suggestions for Par-
> ents."
> When his third child arrived, he quit lecturing altogether
> (Rajneesh, 1978, pp. 21–22).

Riddles might be used to reframe situations and to challenge previously rigid ideas or approaches patients have been
using to try to solve their problems. Watzlawick, Weakland,
and Fisch (1974) made one of Erickson's favorite riddles well-
known when they used it as an illustration for their concept
of reframing. The puzzle is this: Connect these nine dots with
four straight lines without lifting your pen from the paper (see
Figure 1). The solution is included at the end of the chapter
(see Figure 3).

Another favorite Erickson riddle was his challenge to design
an orchard which had ten trees, five straight rows and four
trees in a row. (See Figure 4 at the end of the chapter for the
solution.) (Also see Erickson & Rossi, 1979, p. 342.)

These riddles were usually used to challenge students and

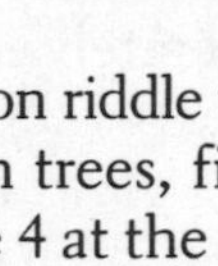

Figure 1

patients to go beyond old frames of reference, to look at things from a new perspective (for more on this topic, see Chapter 6 on Framing Interventions). Erickson would hand people a sheet that had the number 710 or 7105 on it. He challenged them to read it every possible different way they could. Most people never thought of turning the paper upside down and reading the number as a word, either "OIL" or "SOIL." In a similar vein, he would challenge people with the statement that they could not even be sure which hand was right and which hand was left. After getting a person to assure him he knew with absolute certainty which was right and which was left, he would ask him to put his left-sided hand behind his back and then say with amusement, "Now which one is left?" The person could only agree that the right hand was left.

The parallel message in these riddles was that the patient could look at problems from a new perspective.

Puns were used to surprise or confuse people, to deliver interspersed or embedded suggestions. For example, "Having that hand lift to your face can be pretty *disarming*, can it not? Well, you never know what your unconscious can come *up* with, do you?"

Stories can be used to suggest new possibilities and to get clients to yield the floor and listen (Wilk, 1985; Zeig, 1980), to evoke abilities (Lankton & Lankton, 1983), to intersperse suggestions (Zeig, 1980), and to accomplish many other purposes.

Metaphor is a literary device which includes simile (something spoken of as "like" or "as" something else, e.g., "cheeks like roses") and analogy (two things that correspond in some way or share some features, e.g., a computer's disk drive is like a tape recorder/player). Anytime one thing is likened to another or spoken of as if it were another thing, metaphor is involved. "We seemed to have reached a *dead end* in this discussion." "Your smile is like the *summer sun*." Such phrases are in common use; in fact, they are so common that we often fail to recognize metaphorical phrases as metaphor. These devices are used to *cast a different light* (another metaphor) on the subject. We know what a dead end is when we are traveling along a road, so we can understand the analogy when it is used to characterize a discussion. We have experienced a summer sun, so we can imagine that a smile likened to it would be bright. Metaphor helps us use understandings or experiences we have had already to make sense of new experiences.

The etymological meaning of the word "metaphor" gives a clue to the function of metaphor in Erickson's therapy. The word is derived from the Greek roots *pherein*, meaning "to carry" and *meta*, which means "beyond" or "over." The function of metaphor is to carry knowledge across contexts, beyond its initial context into a new one.

Erickson assumed that people already have the abilities, or know-how, to solve the problems that have been troubling them. They have developed and mastered these abilities in certain contexts, but are not currently using them in the contexts in which the problem occurs. The task of therapy, then, is to transfer this know-how across contexts from the one(s) in which the patient currently has it to the context in which he does not. This is accomplished by using metaphor in its various forms.

What follows is a model for using stories, anecdotes, analogies, trance phenomena, and task assignments as parallel communication and in therapy. The model, called the Class of Problems/Class of Solutions Model, has been useful in making sense of some of Erickson's interventions

CLASS OF PROBLEMS/CLASS OF SOLUTIONS MODEL

After one has determined the presenting problem to be solved in therapy (and this determination may have a profound effect on the course of therapy; see O'Hanlon and Wilk, 1987), the first step in using this model is to derive from the specific presenting problem an abstraction that is a *set* of the kinds of problems that this problem exemplifies. The class of problems is not to be an explanation of the problem (e.g., "to keep the parents from discovering their conflict," or "to get attention," or "secondary gain," etc.); rather, it is to be descriptive. An abstraction that includes the kind of abilities that people have to solve that sort of problem is then devised. From that set of abilities (the class of solutions), a specific intervention is derived. The intervention is a parallel communication and treatment agent for the specific presenting problem. The specific intervention is usually a metaphor of some kind (an anecdote or analogy), a task assignment, an interaction, or one of the trance phenomena. These are designed to access or develop the ability that is needed to solve the problem. See Figure 2 for a graphic representation of this process.

Perhaps the best way to understand the model is to look at examples of its use with some problems. The examples used here are all taken from Erickson's work.

Treating Enuresis (Bedwetting)

Erickson described a number of cases in which he used parallel treatment devices to treat enuresis. The specific problem is bedwetting. The class of problems here might be de-

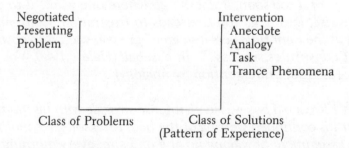

Figure 2. Class of Problems/Class of Solutions Model

scribed as "lack of muscle control." A class of solutions might
be "automatic muscle control." There may be other classes
of problems and classes of solution which could be abstracted
(for example, another class of problems could be "staying
asleep when bladder is full," and a concomitant class of solutions could be "automatically waking up when bladder is full"),
but what we are searching for here are ones that are descriptive and lend themselves readily to interventions. In the cases
that follow, Erickson works towards the goal of automatic
muscle control through such parallel interventions as analogies, task assignments, and interactions.

*A 12-year-old boy was brought to Erickson for bedwetting.
Erickson dismissed his parents and immediately began talking
to the boy about other topics, avoiding a discussion of bedwetting altogether. Upon learning that the boy played baseball
and his brother football, Erickson began to describe the fine
muscle coordination it takes to play baseball compared to the
gross, uncoordinated muscle skills used in football. The boy
listened raptly as Erickson described in some detail all the fine
muscle adjustments his body made automatically in order to
position him underneath the ball and to catch it. The glove
has to be opened up just at the right moment and clamp down
again just at the right moment. When transferring the ball to
another hand, the same kind of fine muscle control was
needed. Then, when throwing the ball to the infield, if one
lets go of it too soon, it doesn't go where one wants it to go.
Likewise, letting go too late leads to frustration. Letting go
just at the right time gets it to go where you want it to go and
that constitutes success . . . in baseball (Haley, 1980, Vol. 3,
pp. 127–130). [Intervention = analogy]*

*A 12-year-old boy was in an intense struggle with his mother
over his continued wetting of the bed. Erickson gave mother
the assignment of waking up at 4 or 5 a.m. every morning to*

check whether her son's bed was wet or dry. If it was dry, she was to go back to bed without waking the boy. If it was wet, she was to get the boy up and have him practice his handwriting (which was very poor) until 7 a.m. Not only was the symptom resolved, but the boy's relationship with his father and his grades at school improved (Zeig, 1980, pp. 106–109). [Intervention = task assignment]

An 11-year-old girl had been cytoscoped so many times for her urinary tract problems that she had lost her ability to control her bladder sphincter. She would wet her pants if she ran or laughed during the day and she wet the bed at night. Her sisters, the neighbor kids and the kids at school had discovered her weakness and took delight in making her wet her pants. She was miserable about the situation. Erickson told her that she already knew how to have dry beds and dry pants. She told him he was wrong. He told her that she already knew but that she did not know that she knew. She was perplexed by that. He asked her in a rather dramatic fashion what she would do if she was sitting on the toilet urinating and a strange man poked his head in the bathroom. She replied that she would freeze. Erickson agreed and told her that this is what she knew that she did not know that she knew. All she had to do, he said, was to use this ability and to practice starting and stopping when she was urinating. She developed her muscles rapidly and was having dry beds and pants within a short time (Rosen, 1982, pp. 113–116; Zeig, 1980, pp. 79–84). [Interventions = interaction + task assignment]

Treating Impotence

As soon as he returned from his honeymoon, a man went to seek Erickson's help. The man explained that during the entire two weeks of the honeymoon he had been unable to get an erection. His bride had taken this very personally and *had been so humiliated that she demanded an annulment. Erickson told the man to bring his wife to the office. When she was there, Erickson told the man that he was to look at his wife and experience anew his feelings of shame and humiliation and that he would do anything to escape from those feelings. It was suggested that he could escape by entering a deep trance in which he would be unable to see anything but his wife. He would then realize that he was losing control of his body and begin to hallucinate his bride in the nude. Next he would start to feel intimate physical contact with his bride that would become more and more exciting. He was reminded that he had succeeded in the office in obtaining an erection and that there would be nothing to stop him from being successful again and again. Consummation occurred that night. Follow-up for over ten years indicated no recurrence of the impotence (Rossi, 1980, Vol. 1, p. 172). [Presenting problem = impotence; class of problems = lack of automatic physiological response; class of solutions = automatic physiological response; intervention = trance phenomena]*

An elderly gentleman sought treatment from Erickson for sexual impotence. The man's wife had died some years before and he had not felt sexual feelings for some time. He had recently started dating a woman and found that he did not respond sexually during their intimate encounters. Erickson reminded him that they had found seeds from Egyptian tombs that had sprouted after 5,000 years. Next Erickson induced a trance with the man and told him that he would not be able to get up out of the chair after he awakened. Then he induced a hand and arm levitation with the man. As the man's hand raised up and touched his hair, Erickson suggested that the man could not stop the levitation and that he could associate the touch of the hair with his hand with the feeling of his lady friend's pubic hair with his penis. Erickson then arranged it so that the hand would not go down until the man had an

*intense feeling of satisfaction (Erickson & Rossi, 1979, pp.
247–267). [Presenting problem = impotence and lack of confidence in ability to respond sexually; class of problems = lack
of automatic physiological response and lack of confidence
in automatic physiological responses; class of solutions =
experience and trust in automatic physiological responses;
intervention = analogy + trance phenomenon (hand levitation)]*

Parallel Treatment of a Husband and Wife

In this last case illustrating the Class of Problems/ Class
of Solutions Model, Erickson provided parallel treatment of
a husband with phantom limb pain (pain experienced where
a leg had been amputated) and his wife with tinnitus (ringing
in the ears). He mainly spoke to the wife, giving her anecdotes
for her tinnitus. At the same time, however, he was providing
a parallel treatment for the husband's phantom limb pain,
since the class of problems and class of solutions are the same
for both problems in this case.

*A man sought Erickson's help for persistent pain in a leg
that had been removed. His wife had also reported that she
had tinnitus. Erickson began the session by telling the couple
about a time when he was traveling around during his college
days and he slept the night in a boiler factory. During the
night, as he slept, he had learned to blot out the sounds in
the factory and by morning he could hear the workers conversing in a normal conversational tone. The workers were
surprised by this, as it had taken them much longer to master
this ability, but Erickson said he knew how quickly the body
could learn. Next Erickson told about seeing a television special the night before about nomadic tribesmen in Iran who
wore layers of clothing in the hot desert sun, but who seemed
very comfortable. During the session he told a number of*

*stories illustrating the ability that people have to become
habituated to any constant stimulus so that they could tune
it out after a while (Erickson & Rossi, 1979, pp. 102–123).
[Presenting problems = phantom limb pain and tinnitus; class
of problems = noxious sensory stimuli; class of solutions =
tuning out noxious sensory stimuli; intervention = anecdotes]*

SYMBOLIC COMMUNICATION

Erickson used *symbolic tasks* to represent certain situations
or emotions concretely for patients. He used *symbolic communication* to speak about certain situations without mentioning them specifically.

*A man who regretted having an affair with the maid wanted
to save the marriage. His wife was furious with him for the
affair and they had separated. In therapy with Erickson, they
decided to stay married. Erickson gave them the assignment
to go home and have the maid pack the husband's clothes in
a suitcase. The maid was then to carry the suitcase out of the
house and throw it in the front yard and bring it back in. The
unpacking and repacking continued until the wife was satisfied that she wanted the husband to move back into the home.
The maid was then fired (Haley, 1985, Vol. 2, pp. 172–173).*

Zeig tells about one of Erickson's cases in which a woman
who had a difficult time getting pregnant finally did, with
Erickson's help. Within the first few years however, the baby
died. For health reasons, the woman could not bear another
pregnancy, so her grief was especially poignant. Erickson advised her to plant a tree and name it after the dead baby girl.
Let us call her Jennifer. In later years, Erickson would come
to visit the woman to sit in the shade of Jennifer (Zeig, 1981).
During a seminar on "Advanced Techniques," Erickson
gave the symbolic analogy of inserting a finger into one's

mouth for use with women with vaginismus (pain when a finger or penis is inserted into the vagina): "Logically, you can put your finger in your mouth and find out for yourself. This far in, you get certain sensations. That far in, you get other sensations. Stick your finger *all the way in* your mouth and you get still different sensations. I haven't talked about the insertion of the penis into the vagina, but I have told her that the lower third of her vagina has different sensations than the middle third, than the upper third. I've also mentioned, without saying it, that there can be an insertion. Now I've talked about the mouth but there's no mistaking. I've talked about mucous membranes. Why shouldn't I talk in a completely safe way and fixate attention?" (Erickson, 1960).

A married woman saw Erickson for the first time and talked on and on about her hair and the difficulty she had parting it correctly. Erickson told the woman that at the end of the interview he would tell her something meaningless. At the end of the interview, he told her that he thought that what she really meant was that she needed to part her hair with a one-toothed comb. She left perplexed. She returned for the next visit wanting to discuss her sexual problems (Haley, 1973, p. 167).

ERICKSON'S USE OF ANALOGIES

. . . you know my tendency to use analogies, and they work. (Erickson, in Haley, 1985, Vol. 2, p. 120)

Erickson: So when you deal with patients, you bear in mind that the unconscious is pretty childlike and pretty direct and pretty comprehensive in its understandings.
Haley: And you typically reach it with analogy?
Erickson: It's the best way, I think. (in Haley, 1985, Vol. 2, p. 123)

As the quotations above indicate, analogies were an important part of Erickson's work and of his use of parallel communication. Although Erickson was known for his stories, far more common in his work are short analogies used to illustrate points or reframe problems for patients and students. As in the Class of Problems/Class of Solution Model, these analogies are aimed at evoking skills or frames of reference to help the patient successfully resolve his or her problem.

Analogies for Pain Control

Erickson's work showed many strategies for successfully controlling and managing the complex phenomenon of pain. Most of these strategies are illustrated by the analogies below. A brief comment following each example indicates the resource that the analogy intends to evoke.

You know how that first mouthful of dessert tastes so very good? And even the second mouthful still tastes good; but by the time you reach the sixty-sixth mouthful, it doesn't taste so good. You have lost the liking for it, and the taste of the dessert has changed in some peculiar way. It hasn't become bad; it has just "died out" in flavor. Now, as you pay attention to these various sensations in your body that you have described to me, I would like you to name the particular sensation that you want me to work on first.

What have I done? I have transformed pain into a single sensation. I have given the patient this analogy of eating the dessert, and of understanding such an analogy, and he can translate it immediately into a lessening of the pain sensation (Rossi, Ryan, & Sharp, 1983, pp. 225–226). [Transformation of sensation; splitting; habituation]

One need only reflect on severely crucial situations of tensions and anxieties to realize that the severest of pain vanishes

*when the focusing of the sufferer's awareness is compelled
by other stimuli of a more intense and life-threatening nature.
From everyday experience, one can think of the mother suffering extremely severe pain to the point where she is all-
absorbed in her pain experience. Yet, she forgets it without
effort and without intention when she suddenly sees her
infant dangerously threatened or seriously hurt. One can think
of men in combat, seriously wounded, but who do not discover
their injuries until hours later when the attack has ceased.
There are numerable such examples common to medical
experience (Rossi, Ryan, & Sharp, 1983, p. 218). [Distraction;
spontaneous pain control]*

*You build up in him the concept of learning how to develop
calluses on the nerves and on the end organs of nerves so that
the nerves become so accustomed to the distressing pruritis
that [the patient as a total personality] doesn't even notice it.
You can also point out the example of the boiler-factory
worker who gets so used to the noise in the factory that he
talks in an ordinary conversational tone of voice to his coworkers, who reply in a normal tone of voice; and they hear
each other despite that infernal din (Rossi & Ryan, 1985, pp.
129–130). [Negative hallucination; tuning out unpleasant stim-
uli]*

*You know you can go to a show, a suspense movie, and
forget about your toothache. You can go to a suspense movie
and forget about your headache. You can have a very pleasant
surprise and forget about your aching corn. Therefore, why
should you think about pain as necessarily treated by anesthesia, as necessarily being treated by analgesia? You've all had
the experience of forgetting a hurt, which means you can treat
pain by inducing amnesia. You can treat pain by distraction
(Rossi & Ryan, 1985, p. 156). [Distraction; amnesia]*

You can take a needle and prick your finger intentionally in order to study the sensation of the needle prick, and you notice how easy it is to localize the needle prick. You feel the prick, but it is a very transient sensation. However, that needle prick would last for a long time if your big brother were pricking you with the needle just to tease you (Rossi & Ryan, 1985, p. 26). [Reframing for different attitudes and circumstances affecting the pain experience]

You see, in organic pain situations you have neurosynapses that are transmitting the pain. Through hypnosis you can spread those synapses apart — like spark plugs jumping a gap — until you have your synapses spread wide apart you get a jumping of the thing. At that point a certain maximal pain stimulation is necessary in order for the person to sense the pain (Rossi & Ryan, 1985, p. 26). [Reframing for increased tolerance of pain]

You think you cannot control pain, and yet every dentist can tell you how easily patients lose their toothaches on the way to the dental office. Every one of you knows that you can have a splitting headache and lose it while watching a suspenseful movie; you lose it not because you have received an intravenous injection for pain, but because your attention has been drawn to more compelling matters — even though that headache was the most compelling matter a few minutes ago (Rossi, Ryan, & Sharp, 1983, p. 183). [Ability to control pain spontaneously; distraction]

Analogies for Evoking Hypnotic Phenomena

Hypnotic phenomena are experiences and skills that are typically shown in trance, such as automatic handwriting, amnesia, analgesia, and anesthesia. In order to ready subjects for the experience of hypnotic phenomena, Erickson used analogies involving common everyday experiences. This not only had the effect of demystifying and normalizing these hypnotic phenomena, but also tended to access these abilities. Following are some examples of analogies for hypnotic phenomena in Erickson's words.

. . . you ought to be able to expect yourself to do automatic writing. Surely you know how to write. Surely you have put on the brake when you have been riding in the back seat of a car; surely you have tensed your mouth and your throat and your vocal cords while listening to a stutterer trying to say a word; surely you have opened your mouth so widely that it was painful to feed that baby that wouldn't open its mouth. You know all of those things; therefore, you can really expect yourself to do automatic handwriting (Rossi & Ryan, 1985, pp. 65–66). [Automatic handwriting]
You can ask a hypnotic subject to develop, let us say, hypnotic deafness, and he will respond: "I can't develop deafness!" Yet we do develop deafness as a matter of course in our everyday lives. We become unaware of certain sounds. The air conditioning is not noticed until it suddenly goes off. You can be reading a paper or a book and your wife speaks to you. Ten minutes later she asks, "Are you going to answer?", and you respond, "Answer what?" How do you develop that deafness? (Rossi, Ryan, & Sharp, 1983, p. 166). [Hypnotic deafness]
Perhaps the best example is amnesia. If I were to ask any one of you to forget some specific item, you would have very great difficulty doing so in your ordinary, waking state. But how many times have you been introduced to a person, been told the person's name, repeated the name, shook hands with the full resolution of remembering that name you have been told; and yet the moment you drop the hand you forget the name? Instant forgetting is as easy in the ordinary waking state, despite your wishes, as it is in the hypnotic state (Rossi, Ryan, & Sharp, 1983, p. 183). [Amnesia]

Other Analogies for Various Purposes

Erickson used analogies for various purposes and to evoke many different skills or frames of reference. Here are several examples, accompanied by explanatory comments, of analogies Erickson used.

The following example is one Erickson used in describing his approach to couples in which an affair has been discovered.

> ... *I see no sense in a rehash. They had all the facts, so did I. The only question was, "Is this the termination of your relationship or is it the beginning of a new one?" If it's termination, period. If it's the beginning of the new, what do you want in this new relationship? In other words, are you moving out of the old house into a new one? If you're moving out, all right, let's not talk about scrubbing the kitchen, the basement, and so on. What do you want in the new house? Now that's a figure of speech, or an analogy, I use quite often. "So you're going to move out of the old house, and leave all of the old furniture there. What kind of view do you want from the new one? It ought to be in a different part of town, with a different view, a different house entirely, with different furniture, different arrangements. Now what do you want in the new house?" (Haley, 1985, Vol. 2, p. 164).*

This last example is from an interview Erickson conducted with a depressed man. Erickson used an analogy to suggest a different frame of reference and a different tact with respect to the depression.

> *Erickson: And what are the particular values in each depression that you have? Because I suspect you have the mistaken idea that depression is wrong.*
>
> *Patient: Well, when I'm depressed I'm, I think, less productive.*

E: Mmmm hmmm. And when you get the rear wheels of your car caught in a ditch, and you can't go ahead in first gear or second gear, third gear, well, I think it's awfully nice to shift into reverse, and then into first, and reverse, and first, and reverse, and first, and rock yourself out of the ditch.
P: Mmmm hmmm.
E: And I think you ought to enjoy it and really rock yourself out of it. And not regret going into reverse. You've learned an awful lot about driving, handling a car (Haley, 1985, Vol. 1, p. 306).

REFRACTION: PARALLEL INDUCTION AND SUGGESTION

Another parallel communication device Erickson used on occasion is that of talking to one person to indirectly put another person into trance or give that second person suggestions. He used this device, which is termed "refraction" (after a term from physics in which light is deflected in two directions), in cases in which it would have been ill-advised or impossible to do a straightforward induction. Erickson would arrange for the person who was to be "secretly" induced to be present in a room in which either a lecture was being given or someone else was being hypnotized. He would then begin his hypnotic induction talk and start to direct his voice toward the unknowing subject while giving suggestions. For example, during a lecture on hypnosis, Erickson might say, "Now some of you may have some experience *going into trance,* and some of you may even have experienced *going into a deep trance.* Most people *close* their *eyes* when they *go into that trance....* " The underlined phrases would be accompanied by significant eye contact from Erickson to the intended subject. He would also start to time his suggestions so that they coincided with the intended subject's behavior (e.g., mentioning inhaling as the subject inhaled). After a time, the suggestions typically had the desired effect and more direct trancework might begin. Alternatively, Erickson might leave it all so circumspect that the person would never realize consciously that a trance induction had taken place.

A related technique was one in which Erickson would start to tell a patient or subject about a friend or previous patient who had been put into trance. In relating what had happened in the previous situation, Erickson would reproduce the trance induction and begin to direct that induction to the present patient or subject. He called this the "My Friend John" technique (Rossi, 1980, Vol. 1, pp. 340–359).

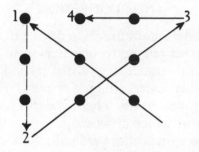

Figure 3. The Solution of the Nine-Dot Problem

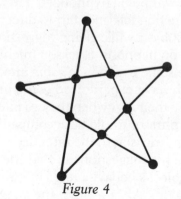

Figure 4

5. *Implication*

> You know what charm is: a way of getting the answer yes without having asked any clear question.
>
> — Albert Camus (1957)

Implication is in some ways the slipperiest of the patterns to discuss. I sometimes say it is like nailing jelly to a tree. When Erickson was asked to analyze his trance inductions or therapy (Erickson & Rossi, 1979; Erickson, Rossi, & Rossi, 1976; Rossi, 1980; Zeig, 1980), he usually mentioned the kinds of things that he wanted to imply with his therapeutic communications, both verbal and nonverbal. However, because different listeners will derive different implications from those communications, this may be more art than science. Erickson often spoke as if he knew what implications patients would take from his communications, which, of course, no one could know for certain. Despite these limitations, implication can be discussed in terms of the techniques that structured Erickson's uses of it.

PRESUPPOSITION

Presupposition is the use of language, actions, and situations that necessarily involve certain antecedents or consequences. One of my favorite examples of presupposition comes from Neil Postman (1976, p. 151), who recounts being asked after a lecture, "Why do you think the extraterrestrials are coming in such large numbers to earth?" If this question

were answered without challenging the presuppositions involved in it, a lot of potential misinformation might be accepted unquestioningly. The question presumes the existence
of extraterrestrials and their numerous visits to earth. The only
question remaining is the reason for the large populations
involved in the visitations. The infamous courtroom question,
asking the defendant, "Have you stopped beating your wife
yet?" is a good example of a presupposition. The only aspect
in question is whether the beating has stopped or not. It is
presumed that it went on at one time. If the question were
answered with a simple yes or no, without challenging the
presupposition, an innocent person might appear guilty. Erickson used presupposition to sneak assumptions and implications past patients. The things he implied were, of course,
therapeutically beneficial for the patient, not for the therapist's
personal gain or satisfaction.

The easiest technique of implication to discuss is *linguistic
presupposition*, in which language is used to imply or presume
something that is therapeutically helpful. Erickson was talking
to a woman who thought she was not very attractive. He told
her about a tribe in Africa in which the women stretch their
lips with plates until they are quite enlarged. Then he said,
"And do you know that the men in that tribe think those are
beautiful, and they're astonished that American men would
consider the kind of lips that you have as beautiful" (Haley,
1985, Vol. 1, p. 20). Here he conveyed the idea that she had
beautiful lips, but said it in such an indirect and impersonal
way that it was difficult for her to consciously recognize or
resist it.

Here is another example of a seemingly simple, innocuous
sentence which concealed several implications through linguistic presupposition. Erickson reported (Rossi, Ryan, &
Sharp, 1983, p. 185) that he said to many patients as they
entered his office, "Please do not go into a trance until you
have seated yourself comfortably in the chair."

Following is an excerpt from a trance induction that Erickson did with a demonstration subject:

MHE: When do you think that your eyes will close?
Subject: I don't know.
MHE: Before or after your hand touches your face? . . .
they're blinking . . . close your eyes now, that's right (Erickson, 1960).

Erickson discussed implication in a lecture on hypnosis by giving an example and pointing out how most people would accept the verbal presupposition unquestioningly: "'And now do you mind letting your hand levitate, slowly at first?' . . . Slowly at first. And what does that imply? Well, rapidly later! A person doesn't try to analyze what you said" (Rossi, Ryan, & Sharp, 1983, p. 242).

A case example from Erickson's work illustrates this use of implication as the main treatment technique that resulted in a reorientation and resolution of the presenting problem.

A woman with an allergy to the sun kept going out into the sunlight, despite warnings from her physicians. She would break out with a severe rash after exposure to the sun, yet she kept sunning herself. While she slept, she would then damage herself scratching at the rash. Her doctors thought she was just too stubborn. She sought Erickson's help in the matter and he put her in a trance and suggested that she enjoy as much of the sunlight as she wished. She was to go home and lie down for an hour or two after the session and let her unconscious mind think over what that meant. The next time she went out into the sun, she wore a wide-brimmed hat and long sleeves. Her rash promptly cleared up (Erickson & Rossi, 1981, pp. 12–13).

Another case again involves implication as the primary

intervention, which, while it didn't resolve the presenting problem, facilitated the therapy:

A colleague referred a rebellious teenager to Erickson. Erickson listened quietly to the boy's story and then said, simply, "I don't know how your behavior will change." This one statement initiated important changes in the boy's life (Erickson, Rossi, & Rossi, 1976, p. 61).

Finally, another example of linguistic presupposition shows the subtle implications that Erickson often used in treatment:

A dentist's wife developed TMJ (a muscle joint problem in the jaw) because she would only chew on the right side of her mouth. She insisted that chewing on the left side hurt. There was nothing physically wrong with her left side. Erickson told her that she should continue to chew only on her right side of her mouth and that if food should get on the left side, she should "haul it back over" to the right side. That phrase implied that she would get food on the left side of her mouth. She soon started eating on both sides of her mouth (Erickson, 1960).

ILLUSION OF ALTERNATIVES

Erickson often called this technique the "double bind," but a true double bind would mean "cured if you do, cured if you don't" and there are few such magical interventions in Erickson's or others' work. Unfortunately, patients have this disturbing habit of not following therapy theory very closely. The illusion of alternatives technique, however, is useful in creating the expectation and implication of positive change in therapy.

Essentially, the technique involves offering the patient two or more choices within a restricted range. Whatever choice the patient makes among the alternatives offered will lead in the desired direction. For example, a patient could be given a task assignment and asked whether he would like to do the assignment once or twice in the interval between sessions. If the patient selects either alternative, it increases the likelihood of the desired result, that of the patient accepting and doing the task assignment. The patient could, of course, refuse to do the task or forget, but the point of this type of intervention is to give the patient the sense that he has chosen the task freely. It is implied that he will agree to do the task; the only question is how often is he going to do it.

THE IMPLIED OPPOSITE

Another type of implication used by Erickson is when one side of a pair of polar opposites is provided and it is left is for the patient to supply the other side. I have termed this technique "the implied opposite." Here are some cases which illustrate its use.

A patient of some dentists in training with Erickson could readily develop a trance, could get glove anesthesia (hypnotic numbing of the hand and part of the arm), but was not successful at the usual procedure of transferring the anesthesia to his mouth and jaw for painless dental work. Erickson suggested that they have him develop an extra hyperesthesia (extreme sensitivity) in his left hand. They did this and the patient spontaneously developed an oral anesthesia, which allowed the dental work to proceed (Rossi, Ryan, & Sharp, 1983, pp. 34-35; Erickson & Rossi, 1976, pp. 77-78).

A patient who had seen Erickson for some time demanded hypnosis, despite the fact that Erickson told him that it wasn't suitable for his situation. Erickson started an induction and continued through the session, while the man continually interrupted to criticize Erickson's efforts. When Erickson stopped the hypnotic work about ten minutes before the session

was over, the man claimed that he was not hypnotized be-
cause he could remember every word that Erickson had said.
Erickson replied that of course the man could remember
everything that was said here because he was here in the
office. Erickson repeated this several times and said he would
prove that the man had been in trance at the next appoint-
ment. Meeting the man in the waiting room before the next
session, Erickson showed that the man had developed an
amnesia outside the office for everything that had occurred
during the previous session and discovered that he could only
regain his memory while in the office (Rossi & Ryan, 1985,
pp. 59–62).

This next case gives an example of Erickson's sense of play
in therapy, as well as the utilization of obvious associations.

A couple came to therapy with Erickson. They had been
married less than a month and the husband was insisting on
a divorce due to the "outrageous behavior" of his bride. Erick-
son accused the man of being a coward and ordered him to
shut up while his bride talked. The woman gave an account
of their sexual relationship, which had to be done according
to the husband's rather stringent standards of what constituted
proper lovemaking. The lights had to be off, the curtains had
to be drawn tightly and she was to wear a nightie during the
sex act. He would not kiss her or touch her in any way except
to insert his penis in her vagina. The husband said that breasts
were for babies only and served utilitarian purposes.
Erickson told the man that his sympathies were with the
wife and that the man probably wouldn't like what Erickson
said. Therefore he was to sit there and listen with his jaws
clenched and his arms folded while Erickson discussed in some
detail with the wife how a husband ought to approach sex with
his wife and how she, as a healthy female, ought to enjoy it.
Erickson then pointed out that people have a tendency to

give pet names to things. They name their guns "Old Betsy,"
their boats "Stay-Up," and their cabins "Do-Come-In." He
suggested that the husband ought to come up with pet names
for his wife's breasts, since he loved her. Erickson suggested
that her twins really ought to have names that rhymed. If the
husband did not name them by the next session, Erickson
would name the first and the husband would be stuck with
naming the second, which would immediately come to the
man's mind. At the second session, the wife reported that her
husband's sexual behavior had been more flexible, but that
he had vowed he would never name the twins. Erickson then
christened the right breast "Kitty." Six months later Erickson
got a Christmas card from them, signed with both their names
and K. and T., along with a note from the wife relating the
great improvement in their sex life and relationship (Haley,
1973, pp. 162–164).

Here Erickson also utilized the man's compulsiveness to
"force" him to change. (See Chapter 2 for a discussion of
utilization.)

THE IMPLIED PREREQUISITE

This type of implication involves getting the patient to
commit to doing something that will involve doing something
else. This something else is therapeutically beneficial and will
be accomplished as the task is completed, but in a way which
may not be immediately apparent to the patient. Erickson
suggested getting hospitalized patients to agree to give the
therapist a recipe or some plant bulbs from their garden when
they return home. When they agree to this, they usually do
not recognize the inadvertent way that they have agreed to
get out of the hospital and go home (Rossi & Ryan, 1985, pp.
187–188).

In another example, from the videotape, "The Artistry of

Milton H. Erickson" (Lustig, 1975), Erickson's demonstration subject comes out of trance to find that she cannot move her hand, as it is still levitated and dissociated from the hypnotic work. Erickson talks with her for a time and then asks her to move his wheelchair over a bit. As she stands up to do this, she finds that she can and does move her hand. Erickson had arranged a situation in which she would discover her ability to move her hand as a prerequisite to moving his wheelchair.

THE IMPLIED RESULT

With this type of implication a patient is told to do something which will lead to some desirable result that may not be immediately apparent in the task. For example, Erickson treated a woman who had a scar on her face that she constantly covered with her hands because it embarrassed her. He persuaded her to go out on a date with one of his students and told her to carry two handbags. Of course, this prevented her from concealing her scar and she quickly discovered that her date was not horrified by her appearance (Rosen, 1982, pp. 64–65).

Erickson used this type of implication with a wife who continually interrupted her husband in the session, even though Erickson had asked her to stop doing so. He asked the wife to take out a tube of lipstick and hold the tip so that it just barely touched her lips. He then asked her to observe with interest how her lips wanted to move as he asked her husband questions (Haley, 1973, p. 227). The logical result of this maneuver was for the wife to remain silent while the husband talked. It is hard to speak clearly with lipstick touching your lips.

6. *Framing Interventions*

> Discovery consists of seeing what everybody has seen
> and thinking what nobody has thought.
>
> —Albert Szent Gyorgyi

Reframing is the therapeutic technique in which a new meaning is associated with facts which previously had other meanings. According to Watzlawick, Weakland, and Fisch (1974, p. 95) "to reframe . . . means to change the conceptual and/or emotional setting or viewpoint in relation to which a situation is experienced and to place it in another frame which fits the 'facts' of the same concrete situation equally well or even better, and thereby changes its entire meaning." The domain of framing interventions is expanded here to include both reframing (providing an alternate frame or meaning for a situation) and deframing (abolishing or casting doubt on current frames or meanings).

Various writers (mainly in the strategic and family therapy fields) have discussed the subject of reframing previously. While these interpretations have been primarily based on or inspired by Erickson's work, explicit procedures and guidelines for understanding Erickson's use of this type of intervention and for creating frame interventions in clinical work have not been thoroughly discussed. The area as a whole seems not to have been very explicitly defined either, resulting in some confusion of the technique with other types of interventions, such as paradoxical interventions and binds.

In this chapter, therefore, an attempt will be made to define and clarify framing interventions through discussion of: (1) the distinction between facts and meanings; (2) the elements of frames; (3) the elements of added meanings; and (4) the distinction between deframing and reframing.

FACTS VS. MEANINGS

Facts are limited to sensory-based observations and descriptions, what actually happens or has happened that can be perceived by our senses.

Meanings are interpretations, conclusions, and attributions that are derived from or related to the facts of the matter. This area will be discussed further in the following sections.

ELEMENTS OF FRAMING

People create frames (or added meanings) from the raw data of sensory experience with the dual processes of "splitting" and "linking" (see Chapter 3). These two operations, taken together, can generate all the elements of meanings that are added to the facts to make up the frame.

ELEMENTS OF ADDED MEANINGS

What follows is a listing and discussion of the various elements of added meanings.

1) *Attributions.* This involves assigning some quality, characteristics or relationship to data. Varieties include:
   a) Causal attributions — claims of cause or affect (e.g., "She made me mad," or "I can't because of my background.")
   b) Attributions of intentions, motivations, purpose and function — claims of reasons "behind" actions and experience (e.g., "He does that just to bug me," or "I must want to punish myself.")

    c) Attributions of personality traits (characterization) — claims of internal psychological or emotional qualities to people (e.g., "He is lazy," or "I think I'm insane.")

    d) Attributions of internal experience to others — often called "mind-reading" — claiming knowledge of someone else's feelings, thoughts or experience (e.g., "He's angry," or "I know you're sitting there judging me.")

2) *Classifying and grouping.* This involves categorizing, joining, and distinguishing the data:

    a) Classification — assigning an element to a class of elements (e.g., "He's an American," or "Positive connotation is one type of reframing.")

    b) Naming — assigning a label to an experience or element (e.g., "That's jazz," or "My name is Bill.")

    c) Generalization — when one or some elements are said to be a larger group or the whole class of elements (e.g., "She's always late," or "If I've told you once, I've told you a million times.")

    d) Characterizing adjectives — assigning some quality to some experience (e.g., "That was a bright idea," or "That was an inefficient way of doing that.")

    e) Equivalences — one experience is said to be identical to another (e.g., "Love is never having to say you're sorry," or "Silence is an admission of guilt.")

    f) Linking — two or more elements are said to be associated (e.g., "Those dishes go together," or "This is just like my last breakdown.")

    g) Splitting — drawing boundaries and sequences (e.g., "He hit me first," or "It's the first day of spring.")

3) *Evaluations* — assigning a value or judgment on the worth or importance of something or someone (e.g., "That's not important right now," or "It was a valuable experience for me.")

4) *Conclusions* (or *implication* or *significance*) — drawing

a conclusion about the meaning or implication of an experience (e.g., "His presence in therapy indicates that he is committed to the marriage.")

a) Predictions — claiming knowledge of the future (e.g., "He'll never amount to anything," or "She's going to experience that grief sooner or later.")

5) *Metaphor.* These are images or phrases used to describe or communicate experience in a non-literal way.

a) Analogies — when one thing is likened to another (e.g., "Your son is really like a husband," or "I feel like I'm in a deep, dark hole.")

b) Metaphorical frames — when an image is implicit in a description (e.g., "My mind was racing a mile a minute. I was a million miles away," shows the "thoughts as travelers" frame.)

c) Metaphor — when a story (characterized by descriptions of action and a beginning, middle, and end) is told (e.g., "Once a man wanted to find out whether computers could think like humans. So he gathered all the best computer programmers and equipment around him and set them to the task of answering the question. When preparations were complete, he typed in the question: DO YOU COMPUTE THAT YOU CAN THINK LIKE A HUMAN BEING? After some time, the printer began typing, THAT REMINDS ME OF A STORY . . . ")

DEFRAMING AND REFRAMING

When patients report their complaints to therapists, they report both the facts and the added meanings. If the therapist challenges (either directly or indirectly) the meanings patients associate with the situation without providing a new frame, this is *deframing.* Patients are left to create or discover alternative meanings for themselves or to accept the situation without any particular meanings. If the therapist provides a new or alternative frame or meaning to the situation (again, either directly or indirectly), this is *reframing*.

By altering the elements of added meanings that patients offer with the facts of their situation (by either challenging and casting doubt upon current frames or by providing alternative frames), the therapist can either provide a new frame that is more amenable to therapeutic interventions or abolish the "problem" frame so that there is no longer any "problem" to solve.

CASE EXAMPLES AND ANALYSES

Following are some case examples, with commentary included within the example in brackets to show the use of this framework:

Erickson saw in therapy a single nurse whom he had observed had very large buttocks and also a love for children. He reports that he said to her, "I KNOW you've got the biggest fanny in creation. I KNOW you don't like it, but it IS yours. And you like children, therefore you'd like to get married, have children of your own. [Reframing, mind-reading: attributions of what she likes and wants] And you're afraid that great big fanny of yours is a barrier . . . that's your error. [Deframing, challenging causal attribution: big fanny does not cause you not to be married and have children] You haven't read the Song of Solomon. You SHOULD have read your Bible. The pelvis is mentioned as the cradle of children. [Reframing, reclassifying: pelvis is assigned to the class of cradles of children] The man who will want to marry you will not see a great big fat fanny . . . he'll see a wonderful cradle for children." [Reframing, new equivalence: big fat fanny = cradle for children; new prediction: men won't notice big fanny, only cradle] Men who want to father children DO want a nice cradle for the child (Gordon & Meyers-Anderson, 1981, pp. 67–69). [Re-framing, new significance and evaluation: you've got a nice cradle that men who want to father children will want]

While a patient of Erickson's was in a hypnotic age regression, she told about an experience that was somewhat traumatic for her, in which she broke a window. He asked her whether she enjoyed it and she said she was shocked. Erickson said, "It's nice to learn what a shock is" (Grinder, DeLozier, & Bandler, 1977, p. 145). [Reframing, new evaluation and implication: shock is nice and you learned something]

A woman executive sought therapy from me because she lost her voice (or it became very hoarse and shaky) when she spoke in meetings. She initially stated that it was related to "low self-esteem." When asked how she knew this difficulty was related to her speaking difficulty, she seemed a bit surprised and mentioned that she had been to a hypnotist who suggested that they work on her self-esteem as a way of getting over the problem. I replied, after gathering more information, that as far as I could tell, there was no connection between her self-esteem and this voice difficulty [deframing, abolishing causal attribution: self-esteem does not cause voice difficulty]. Furthermore, with the evidence she had provided, in addition to her appearance and demeanor (she dressed quite well and spoke articulately and confidently), I saw little evidence of a lack of self-esteem. On the contrary, she seemed to have a good level of self-esteem. I asked her if she felt badly about herself. She replied that, no, she did not, but had assumed this was a problem after seeing the hypnotist (with no results) and reading many self-help books. I suggested we get on with matters more relevant to her concerns. She readily agreed. [Deframing, no conclusion: no conclusion of low self-esteem needs to be made]

A mother in therapy with her daughter wasn't ensuring that her diabetic daughter took her shots or gave urine samples

*when she needed to manage her diabetes. The therapist sug-
gested that the mother imagine she was a nurse and needed
to take care of her patient, charting her progress and reviewing
the charts with the doctor. Mother was given a nurse's uniform
and told she was not now Mrs. Robins, but Nurse Robins. The
shots, testing and charting were now handled as they needed
to be (Madanes, 1984, pp. 7–20). [Reframing, new analogy:
mother as nurse]*

   *A woman who had been a patient of Erickson's brought her
eight-year-old daughter to see him. The girl had decided that
she hated herself and everyone else because she was unhappy
with her freckles, for which she was teased unmercifully by
the other children at school. She entered the office angrily.
The first thing Erickson said to her was, "You're a thief! You
steal!" She angrily disagreed with him, but he said he could
prove it. She challenged him to prove it and he said that he
knew where she was when she stole. She was in the kitchen
reaching up to the cookie jar containing cinnamon cookies,
cinnamon buns and cinnamon rolls and it had spilled all over
her face. (Erickson had learned from her mother that about
the only thing she liked these days was cinnamon.) He called
her Cinnamon Face. They shared a laugh at this joke and
established a relationship which led to a change in her attitude
to her freckles. She was now proud of her nickname, Cinnamon Face (Rosen, 1982, pp. 152–154). [Reframing, new
evaluation and linking: freckles as humorous and pleasant;
reframing, new name: Cinnamon Face]*

   *A student of Erickson's returned early from his honeymoon
on the verge of a marital dissolution because he was not able
to get an erection with his new bride. She was very insulted.
Erickson saw the couple together and suggested that the
groom had paid his bride the ultimate compliment. The perplexed couple was told that the man apparently found his
wife's beauty so overwhelming that he was temporarily unable*

to respond (Haley, 1985, Vol. 2, pp. 118–119). [Reframing, new function: Instead of not appreciating his wife, his behavior was showing appreciation]

A businessman with a dependency on cocaine and Percodan, which he had used to treat the severe headaches he had had since he was seven years old, was challenged by Erickson about his honesty in business. He defended himself quite vehemently, protesting his honesty. Erickson then confronted him on the dishonesty of keeping a seven-year-old boy's headache. The man was angry at Erickson for insisting on this point, but when he went home he noticed he had no headache. The man returned and confessed that Erickson had been correct; he must have been hanging on to that little boy's headaches. He no longer took the drugs and no longer had a headache (Haley, 1973, pp. 258–259). [Reframing, splitting and linking: it was not his headache, but that of a seven-year-old boy; new implication: keeping the headache was dishonest]

7. *Ambiguity*

Erickson often behaved and communicated with patients and students in an ambiguous manner, leaving his meaning open to many interpretations. When I got that first phone call from him to arrange a visit, his question, "Don't you think you ought to survey the territory before you decide to take the job?" did not lend itself to ready clarification. I recently thought about another possible meaning for that vague question, even though it has been almost ten years since I heard those words. Erickson was a master at creating ambiguous, yet compelling, communications. I sometimes describe talking with him as like being in the Twilight Zone. It seemed to me as if one never knew exactly what the rules were when one was in Erickson's presence, as if all the ordinary rules were suspended and new ones were in effect. There was, at the same time, though, a sense that one was supposed to be responding in some way or doing something. The usual social cues that ordinarily give hints as to what that something might be were not clear or were absent altogether.

What was the purpose of this ambiguity? One purpose was to motivate patients to make their own meanings, thereby customizing therapeutic interventions and communications. Most of us do not tolerate this ambiguity well and are highly motivated to make some order out of the chaos. Since the clues were not forthcoming from Erickson, patients were thrown back on their own resources to resolve this dilemma. Consistent with his positive view of people's abilities, Erickson was confident that once the context was provided, patients would find their own solutions.

The particular patient's response to ambiguity can also provide valuable information and direction to the therapist who does not want to impose his values and ideas on the patient.

THE CONFUSION TECHNIQUE

Hans Eysenck, the British psychologist, tells a charming story (1957, pp. 32–33) about a friend of his who had to hypnotize a shell-shocked French soldier. As the soldier spoke no English, the friend gave the suggestions in French, in which he was none too proficient. Instead of telling the subject that his eyes were closing, he inadvertently told the man that his nostrils were closing. Eysenck reports that it seemed to make no difference, since the man went into a good trance anyway. Erickson might have another view of the matter, however, and consider this to be a good example of the use of the "confusion technique."

The confusion technique was a method Erickson developed for overwhelming the subject's conscious, rational thinking in order to facilitate induction. In his article on the subject (Rossi, 1980, Vol. 1, pp. 258–291), Erickson relates two incidents that led to the development of this technique. One involved a lab partner of Erickson's who bragged to his classmates that he was going to get Erickson to perform the difficult and tedious part of the upcoming experiment. Erickson, however, got wind of the scheme, and when the time for the experiment arrived, Erickson said intently to his partner, "That sparrow really flew to the right, then suddenly flew left, and then up, and I just don't know what happened after that." While his partner stared at him in bewilderment, Erickson gathered up the equipment for the easy part of the experiment and set to work. His partner unthinkingly took the rest of the material and went to work, only later realizing that he was doing the difficult part.

Another pivotal incident occurred while Erickson was bracing himself against the wind one day. A man came around the corner and bumped into him. Before the man could speak a word, Erickson glanced at his watch and said, "It's exactly 10 minutes of two," when in fact it was around 4:00. Erickson then walked off, leaving the bewildered man there. From these early pranks, Erickson realized that a trance-like response had been elicited from both people in response to the non sequiturs. He decided to experiment with this as a deliberate induction technique and found that it worked very well.

Erickson used not only words but also actions to provide ambiguity or confusion in therapy.

A Mormon woman who was dying of cancer was seen in her home by Erickson for help with her severe pain. She reported that she did not believe that hypnosis could help her with the kind of pain she had. Her 18-year-old daughter was present while Erickson was talking to the woman. Erickson told the woman that he understood her skepticism, but that "seeing is believing." Erickson turned to the daughter and explained to her that she could take as much time as she wanted to go into a trance, but that, despite the fact that she had probably never been in a trance before, she would probably want to develop one as quickly as possible. She rapidly went into trance and Erickson instructed her to lose all feeling in her body. Then Erickson lifted the girl's skirt and slapped her hard on the thigh. She reported that she could not feel it at all. The daughter was systematically taught to dissociate various parts of her body and the mother learned while watching. Not only was this a parallel treatment of the mother through the daughter, but it was such a confusing, ambiguous action that mother was thoroughly entranced and challenged by seeing her daughter treated thus. Was Erickson a dirty old

*man? Was this hypnosis? The confusion helped to reorient
the woman to a trance and to the possibility of pain control.
(Haley, 1973, pp. 306–310)*

Erickson wrote about several nonverbal confusion techniques that he used to induce trances. One was the "handshake induction." This was described in detail by Erickson in
several settings (Rossi, 1980, Vol. 1, pp. 331–339; Erickson,
Rossi, & Rossi, 1976, pp. 108–111), but here it will be summarized by saying merely that Erickson interrupted a normal
handshake and turned it into an evocation of arm catalepsy
and hypnosis by making his touches and his gaze very ambiguous. Subjects lacked the normal social cues for interpreting this strange behavior and usually responded by entering
a trance and developing catalepsy.

There seem to be three major elements to a confusion
technique in therapy: (1) out-of-context remarks or behavior,
(2) remarks or behavior that lend themselves to two or more
interpretations, and (3) a process of overwhelming patients'
or subjects' conscious processing capabilities. The first category, out-of-context remarks and behavior, has already been
discussed; the next two categories are considered below.

Remarks or Behavior That Lend Themselves
to Two or More Interpretations

In their 1975 book about Erickson's hypnotic language
patterns, Bandler and Grinder specified many types of words
that can facilitate hypnotic inductions. The primary characteristic of these words is that they do not specify any particular
meaning. In most counseling, specificity and concreteness are
prized as good therapeutic skills, but in Erickson's work, especially his hypnosis, there is an emphasis on almost the exact
opposite. The words that Erickson used in most of his communication are what could be called "empty words"—"empty"

because they are devoid of specific reference and meaning. These empty words are not specified as to time, place, person, thing or action. The client or subject can fill in his own meaning because the therapist or hypnotist has not supplied one.

A colleague from England (Phil Booth) came to the U.S. to study with John Weakland, a former student of Erickson's who is now a prominent therapist in his own right. When Weakland asked Phil how he got there, Phil was not sure whether he was being asked how he physically got to John's office (e.g., by plane, car, etc.) or how he became interested in Weakland's work. When he asked for clarification, Weakland's response was, "Whatever level you want to fly at!" (Booth, 1984) This seemed typical of Erickson's ambiguity. Ask patients and students to respond, but leave the level of response up to them.

Erickson was doing some hypnotherapy with a woman and asked her to reexperience a traumatic childhood experience. She experienced a time when she received a spanking for breaking a window. Erickson suggested that she reexperience the spanking, but he did it in such an ambiguous way that it was not clear whether he was going to give it to her or she should imagine it. Erickson asked her, "How would you like another spanking?" She replied, "I'd want to know who's going to give it to me?" Erickson, never one to be pinned down, said, "You want to know. You'll know when your eyes are closed . . ." (Grinder, DeLozier, & Bandler, 1977, p. 157).

Other types of empty words include idioms (e.g., "You can *breathe easier* knowing that your unconscious is working for you," might be very useful for an asthma patient), and puns (e.g., "And the images can *come more easily* as time goes on," might be a useful phrase to use with a non-orgasmic woman).

Overwhelming Conscious
Processing Capabilities

In this approach, so many confusing verbalizations are provided by the hypnotist/therapist that the subject/patient gives up trying to consciously process all that is being communicated. Zeig (1984) gives a formula for constructing such confusing verbalizations. He suggests that the hypnotist start with two opposite concepts, like wrong and right, and juxtapose them, sometimes adding two other concepts into the mix. In the following example, Zeig, uses the example of a small child who opens a present by mistake. Zeig launches into a confusing series of statements which is very difficult for the listener to follow consciously.

> . . . and sometimes a child makes the right mistakes for the wrong reasons, and sometimes a child makes the wrong mistakes for the right reasons, and some of those mistakes that are right now can be wrong at a later time, and some of the wrong mistakes now can be made right at a later time, and some of the understandings now that can be misunderstood at a later time, can only be understood at a far later time. . . . (Zeig, 1982)

Another technique Erickson often used was to speak in ungrammatical sentences and phrases and to leave phrases unfinished. This was intended again to confuse and distract the patient so that he would be more open to new experiences and direction from the therapist. In an induction Erickson said, " . . . just waiting . . . and you know why I'm waiting for. . . . That's right" (Grinder, DeLozier, & Bandler, 1977, pp. 122–123). What is one to make of such a communication?

Elements of Erickson's Therapy and Hypnosis

8. Phases of Erickson's Therapy

While it would be a distortion to give a formula for Erickson's therapy, I offer here a general framework for the sequence and structure of his work.

GAINING RAPPORT/ENGAGING

A long-standing tradition in hypnosis calls for the hypnotist to "gain rapport," to develop a feeling of trust and understanding with the subject. Likewise, in therapy the development of rapport, trust, empathy, and mutual understanding has been emphasized. Through Erickson's work with hypnosis, he developed ways of rapidly gaining the trust and cooperation of patients, both with hypnosis and in his nonhypnotic work. This rapid development of rapport paved the way for Erickson's development of brief therapy. If it took one several months or years to develop rapport in therapy, therapy must of necessity be long-term. Erickson occasionally did one-session therapy and, even in longer cases, often made interventions in the first session.

GATHERING INFORMATION

Erickson's work shows that he continued his assessment process throughout the course of therapy. Most therapists do a diagnostic assessment at the outset of therapy and base the rest of their interventions on this initial diagnosis. Erickson rarely used psychiatric diagnoses to describe patients and considered them too broad a description on which to base therapy. He seemed more interested in discovering patients' patterns and styles of responsiveness. What would they respond to?

BYPASSING OR INTERFERING WITH SELF-IMPOSED LIMITATIONS AND BELIEFS

Erickson thought that patients had problems because they acted and thought in rigid patterns. One of his therapeutic goals was to break up their rigid beliefs about their problems. He believed that people limited themselves unnecessarily. Confusion, as discussed in Chapter 7, was a major tool used to bypass and interfere with patients' and subjects' self-limiting beliefs. Reframing, as discussed in Chapter 6, was another of these tools. Pattern intervention, even though it mainly involves intervening in rigid patterns of behavior, can also have the effect of challenging patients' self-imposed limitations. The main point of using hypnosis was to bypass conscious, limiting beliefs.

Another method Erickson used for bypassing conscious limitations was shock and surprise. He would do or say something so unexpected that patients would be at a loss to explain it or respond in their usual ways. One particular case of Erickson's stands as a good example of this use of shock and surprise.

A man and a woman who were both college professors had met, fallen in love and married. They had been married for some years and had as yet had no children. They sought Erickson's help because they had both been thoroughly checked and no physiological explanation for the infertility could be found. They suspected that it was psychologically or emotionally based. They were very rational people and had engaged in what they described as "marital union with full physiological concomitants every night and every morning for procreative purposes." They were extremely embarrassed and formal when describing the rigid rituals that they had developed in order to satisfy their "philoprogenitive desires."

Erickson told them that he had a treatment for them, but that he did not know whether they were strong enough to bear it. It would be "shock treatment." It would not be electrical shock, but rather psychological and emotional shock treatment. They were to sit in his waiting room and discuss it. After some time, they appeared back in his office and announced that they were ready for whatever it might take to cure the infertility.

Erickson told them that they were to hang onto their chairs tightly. He would tell them something and then they were to leave the office. They were not to speak another word to him or to each other until they were home. Erickson repeated in their stilted formal language the problem, that they had repeatedly engaged in marital union with full physiological concomitants every morning and every evening, but that now they were to go home and "fuck for fun and pray to the devil that she doesn't get knocked up for at least three months." The stunned couple were ushered out of the office and reported later that they had driven home in silence. Upon arriving home, they found that they could not wait to get to the bedroom, where they did indeed "fuck for fun." The woman was pregnant within three months (Haley, 1973, pp. 164–166).

Erickson reported that he was reluctant to publish the case and that when he spoke about it to a medical audience, even these "scientific" medical doctors were shocked by the language. I think, however, that Erickson got rather a thrill out of shocking his audience and readers.

EVOKING ABILITIES
AND/OR MOTIVATION

The topic of evoking abilities has been covered in some
detail in Chapter 4 in the sections on analogies and the Class
of Problems/Class of Solutions Model. In this section, Erickson's use of other techniques to access motivation and resources will be examined.

Erickson had an uncanny ability to create an atmosphere
in which people could get access to the competence or motivation they needed to resolve their problems.

*An example of evoking competence is a case of Erickson's
in which a boy blocked completely on reading. He was 11 years
old, but every year the teachers would start him again on a
first grade reader. Erickson learned that he had taken a
summer vacation on the West Coast. Erickson provoked an
argument with the boy by insisting that Los Angeles was 750
miles away and that Spokane was 350 miles away. The boy
knew differently. Erickson got out the map to check. Erickson
started looking for Spokane around Salt Lake City, but the
boy corrected him and found it on the map near Portland.
After a series of mistakes like that, the boy gradually got
better and better at reading the names on maps. Erickson
mentioned that he was a member of an automobile club that
would provide free maps and literature for planning trips. The
boy persuaded his father to join the club and got a lot of maps
and literature for planning the next family vacation. He read
it all and advised his father on the routes they should take and
what sights they should see. The boy joined his classmates
in reading at the appropriate level when school started in the
fall that year (Haley, 1985, Vol. 3, 126–127).*

Another example of accessing competence and motivation
is provided in the following case. Erickson seemed to be willing

to do just about anything, even have patients get very angry at him, if it would facilitate the therapy.

A woman from another state brought her husband to be treated by Erickson. He was a very proud man who had suffered an incapacitating stroke. Before his stroke, he had been an independent man who had run his own business. After the stroke, he was not able to move much or to talk at all, and he had lost the family business and money to medical bills. He had been hospitalized for over a year in a teaching hospital, where he continually suffered the humiliation of being used as a teaching example of a "hopeless case." A physician had referred them to Erickson, recommending hypnosis as a possible rehabilitation aid. Erickson saw the man's wife first and she told him that her husband was proud and did not like to take orders from anyone. Erickson had the man brought in and proceeded to call him a Nazi Prussian pig (referring to the man's ethnic background) who was content to lie in a charity bed. He then told the man that he was going to have his wife bring him in each day for more insults. The man got so angry that he yelled "No!" and struggled out of the room on his own power. Each day the man was brought by his confused wife to Erickson's office, where Erickson insulted him and evoked the reactions that led to the man's recovery of speech and movement. At the end of therapy, the wife was startled to hear her husband tell Erickson that he loved him like a brother (Haley, 1973, pp. 310–313; Rossi, 1980, Vol. 4, pp. 321–327).

BUILDING SKILLS

For the most part Erickson, with his naturalistic approach, seemed to assume that patients had all the resources and experiences they needed to resolve the problems that brought

them to therapy. Sometimes, however, he would evoke potentials to build skills that the patient had not fully developed.

*A good example of this approach is Erickson's work with a
woman called "Ma" (Rossi, 1980, Vol. 1, pp. 197–201), who had
always wanted to learn to read and write, but had never been
able to overcome her block to these goals. She was not allowed
to learn when young and resolved to learn from the age of 16.
At the age of 20 she hit upon the idea of taking in teachers
as boarders and having them teach her to read and write. Her
boarders and later her children all tried to teach her, all to no
avail. She would become frightened and go blank when anyone tried to explain reading and writing to her.*

*At the age of 70, she came in contact with Erickson, still
unable to read. Erickson promised her that she would be
reading and writing within three weeks and that he would ask
her to do nothing that she did not already know how to do.
She was skeptical and intrigued. First he asked her to pick up
a pencil. He told her to pick it up any way, like a baby would.
Next he asked her to make some marks on a paper, any scrib-
bling marks like a baby that can't even write would do. Then
he asked her to make some straight lines, like she would do
on a board when she wanted to saw or like she would in a
garden when she wanted to plant a straight row. She could
make the lines up and down or across or sideways. Then she
was to draw some donut holes and then draw the two halves
of a donut when it is broken in half. Then she was to draw
the two sides of a gabled roof. He continued to instruct her
to make these marks and to practice them. She practiced
although she did not see the relevance of it.*

*Next session Erickson told her that the only difference
between a pile of lumber and a house was that the latter was
merely put together. She agreed to this, but again did not see
the relevance. With Erickson's guidance, she put those marks*

together to make all the letters of the alphabet. When she had
completed that, Erickson let her in on the fact that she had
just learned to write all the letters. Spelling words was merely
a matter of putting letters together. Erickson got her to name
certain words. Gradually he maneuvered her into writing a
sentence and had her name all the words in it. The sentence
read, "Get going Ma and put some grub on the table." When
she said this aloud, she realized it was just like talking. The
translation into reading was then easily made within a three-
week period.

LINKING SKILLS AND ABILITIES TO
THE PROBLEM CONTEXT

During most of Erickson's career the spirit of the times
dictated that therapy was to happen mainly in the therapist's
office and to be centered mainly around the patient's relationship with the therapist. Erickson was more interested in having patients as quickly as possible translate therapeutic gains
to their daily lives. One of the ways he accomplished this goal
was by having patients perform tasks and take actions related
to the problem.

Another way Erickson linked the skills and abilities that had
been evoked to the problem context was by posthypnotic
suggestion. He would suggest that the next time this particular
context or stimulus arose, the patient could respond in this
particular way. For example, if he had accessed relaxation as
a resource for a phobic patient, he would suggest that the next
time the patient was in the presence of the feared object or
situation, he could relax.

A third method for transferring skills to the problem context was to link the problem situation with new associations
through the use of stories or indirect suggestion techniques.
These have been discussed extensively in Chapters 4 and 5.

TERMINATING THERAPY
AND FOLLOW-UP

At times Erickson would not terminate therapy, but would follow a "family doctor" kind of model, seeing people as needed for years. He would even see several generations of a family over the course of many years. This was perhaps a reflection of his view that therapists do not need to take care of every potential problem in therapy. His was a more limited, problem-focused approach for the most part. (Of course, Erickson being Erickson, it should be obvious by now that there were exceptions to this general "rule.")

At other times, he would abruptly terminate therapy, sending patients away and implying that what therapy they had gotten was all they would need. With other patients, he would set a time limit on therapy. This seemed to create an expectation of results within the time frame provided.

Erickson had a nice naturalistic technique of doing follow-up without reminding people of their problems and in a way that made it likely they would stay in contact with him for a number of years. He asked to be put on patients' Christmas card list. So, once a year, he would receive a card with a note and/or a picture of the family giving some indication of the current situation. He also seemed to lack most therapist's reticence to interact socially with patients; his case examples are replete with references to informal follow-up contacts in casual social settings.

9. *Elements of Erickson's Trance Inductions*

PERMISSIVE VS. AUTHORITARIAN INDUCTION APPROACHES

An "Ericksonian" approach to induction can be distinguished from traditional, "authoritarian" or more directive approaches by its use of permissive language. Authoritarian approaches try to bolster the effect of hypnosis by getting the subject to comply with specific suggestions or directives. A permissive approach does not require one particular response or precondition for successful trance, but allows for many possible responses. In this way, many potential issues of resistance and control are bypassed.

Authoritarian approaches typically use two major types of language in suggestions:

1) Attributional—this involves telling subjects what they are experiencing (e.g., "You are deeply in trance," or "You are very relaxed.")
2) Predictive—telling subjects what they are going to experience or do (e.g., "Your arm will lift up to your face," "You will go deeply into trance," or "You'll relax more and more.")

These kind of authoritarian suggestions are all well and good if the subject shows the proper response to the suggestions. There is trouble, however, if the subject does not respond or in fact shows the opposite of the expected response. This difficulty is avoided by the use of permissive language and approaches in an Ericksonian approach.

Permissive language involves using "possibility words" like "can," "might," "could," etc., and giving many options for what the person is and will be experiencing or doing (e.g., "You might be going deeply into trance," "Your right hand could lift to your face, your left hand might lift up, or both hands can remain comfortably on your thighs or something else all together might happen.") Again, this gives the subject a sense of freedom and bypasses potential resistance.

Permissive approaches also validate any experience or response as appropriate. Each experience or response is validated as acceptable and as an adequate link to the desired result (e.g., "If your conscious mind is distracted by the sounds around or your thoughts, your unconscious mind can be more free to help you go into a trance," or [if the hand levitation that was suggested did not occur] "That's fine, your unconscious can make choices that are appropriate for you, and perhaps those hands can develop that weighted or detached feeling that accompanies a more profound trance experience."). I sometimes say that Ericksonian hypnosis is "hypnosis for chickens." It is for those of us who do not have the confidence that the subject will respond exactly as we suggest. The Ericksonian hypnotist arranges it so that neither he nor the subject can fail.

This is not a black and white dichotomy. Most people (Erickson included) use a combination of permissive and authoritarian approaches. As Erickson emphasized again and again, there is no "right" method. The induction must be individualized for the particular subject or patient.

EVOCATION NOT SUGGESTION

A point often unrecognized in discussions of Erickson's hypnotic approaches is that he did not rely on hypnotic *suggestion* as much as on hypnotic *evocation* in induction and treatment. Consistent with his "naturalistic" orientation (discussed in Chapter 1), Erickson assumed that subjects and patients had in their personal history and experience skills that would allow them to develop a trance and trance phenomena (like amnesia, anesthesia, dissociation, etc.) and to resolve their problems. The hypnotherapist's job is to evoke those abilities. This involves creating a context in which the abilities naturally or readily manifest themselves. The elements for evoking these hypnotic abilities are detailed below.

Presupposition

Presupposition is a form of language in which certain ideas or experiences are presumed without ever being directly stated. Perhaps the best known of the types of presuppositions that Erickson used is "the illusion of alternatives" (see Chapters 2 and 5 for other discussions of the technique). The illusion of alternatives is a technique in which several alternatives are offered to the subject. Each of the alternatives offered will lead in the desired direction. So, one could say to a subject: "Would you like to go into a light trance or a deep trance?" "Would you like to go into a trance now or wait until later in the session?" "You can go into a trance with your eyes open or your eyes closed, whatever is more comfortable for you." "You might go in quickly or you might go in more slowly." These are all sentences that have a common presupposition: that you will go into trance sometime in the future. The only questions are: light or deep, sooner or later, eyes open or closed, quickly or slowly. Of course, the subject could, even with these techniques, refuse to go into trance or resist. For the most part, however, subjects are willing to go into a trance — they just do not know how and may experience difficulty in deliberately doing so. The use of this kind of presupposition facilitates this process.

There are other kinds of presuppositions used in an Ericksonian induction, all having the implication that the person will respond in a certain way or have a trance experience. In one of Erickson's inductions, he tells the subject, "Well, Monde, this time, I'd like to have you take your time about going into a trance. I don't want you to go into trance too soon. And you know how easy it is for you. . . . Not quite that fast" (Grinder, DeLozier, & Bandler, 1977, pp. 121–122). Here he has presupposed that she will go into a trance. There is just some discussion about the rate at which she will enter the trance. He also implies that it is easy for her to enter trance.

"Have you ever been in a trance before?" might get you the same verbal response as the question, "Have you ever been in trance?" The implication in the first sentence is that you will go into a trance in the near future. That implication is lacking in the second. Through the use of various sentences that imply that the subject will experience trance sometime in the future, a context — or an expectation — is created in which trance can be easier to attain.

Of course, using presuppositional sentences does not "make" a subject go into trance. It is just one of the elements involved in creating the context for trance.

Contextual Cues

Contextual cues are behaviors, nonverbal communications, settings, lighting, etc., that are either reminders of previous trance experiences or suggestions of a trance context. In my office, I often turn off the overhead fluorescent lights and turn on an incandescent light on my desk before I do a trance induction. This tends to signal to subjects that the context has changed and prepares them for trance. Erickson had a "trance chair" in his teaching seminars that became for the participants a cue; they would go into trance when they sat there after the first induction was performed with a subject in the chair.

One type of contextual cue occurs when the hypnotist alters his usual communication patterns and shifts to his "trance voice" or "trance words." After the first trance, every time that those same voice tones, facial expressions, phrases or words are used, the subject has a cue that this is a "trance context." In listening to tapes of Erickson's demonstrations, one can detect a shift in voice tone and volume that consistently signals the beginning of trance talk.

Likewise, when the subject is instructed to move to a different chair, when the hypnotist turns off a bright overhead light and turns on a dim desk light, etc., the subject is given an indirect suggestion to go into a trance. Whatever elements of the environment or behaviors of the hypnotist have been present at each previous trance experience the subject has observed or experienced serve as powerful cues for future trances.

Nonverbal Matching

Basically, nonverbal matching involves the hypnotist matching his behavior to the subject's behavior. The hypnotist might match his nonverbal behavior to the subject's rhythms, postures, voice qualities, breathing rates, etc. — any ongoing observable behavior. Bandler and Grinder (1975) call this mirroring. This is because the hypnotist mimes or mirrors exactly the subject's behavior. Bandler and Grinder (1975) also discuss a form of matching called cross-mirroring. This is just a fancy term for the hypnotist matching one part of his behavior to some different behavior of the subject. For example, the hypnotist might speak only when the subject exhales, thus matching the subject's behavior, not doing so exactly, but in another form. When the subject's breathing alters, the hypnotist's rate of speaking alters correspondingly. On the exhalation, the hypnotist speaks; on the inhalation, the hypnotist is silent. This has the effect of facilitating rapport between the hypnotist and the subject. It seems to facilitate the acceptance of suggestions. In addition, with the alteration of the usual cadence and rate of the hypnotist's speaking, there is a contextual cue that marks this context as trance. Rarely does one speak in such altered rhythmic ways except in a hypnotic context.

Verbal Matching

Verbal matching has several elements. The first is matching the subject's vocabulary to insure understanding and a development of rapport. If the hypnotist typically uses the word "unconscious," as I usually do, but the subject typically talks about the "subconscious," the hypnotist can adjust his vocabulary to match the subject's.

Another kind of verbal matching is called "descriptive matching." In descriptive matching, the hypnotist basically describes the behavior that the subject shows, in effect operating like a human biofeedback machine. For example, the hypnotist could say to the subject, "Your hands are resting on your thighs." Describing observable behavior and focusing the subject on this aspect of his experience can have the effect of facilitating rapport and building credibility for the hypnotist. The hypnotist is, after all, only telling the subject the truth about his behavior. It also usually has the effect of focusing the subject on only certain aspects of his experience, and this narrowing of the focus of attention can be trance-inducing. Later, for most people in trance, the focus will shift to more internal experience, but initially this focus just on their body, their behavior, and their sensory experience can facilitate trance.

CONFUSION

Erickson seemed to have the idea that people had limiting beliefs that would interfere with the development of trance. These beliefs were maintained by the vigilance of the conscious mind. Erickson used surprise and confusion to bypass such self-imposed limitations, often by giving such complex verbalizations that the subject had trouble following them. Zeig's (1984) formula for the construction of confusion (see Chapter 7) involves picking two sets of polar concepts, like "conscious/unconscious" and "forget/remember," and weaving them together in a constantly changing fashion. For example:

> Your unconscious can forget some things that your conscious mind remembers, but your conscious mind has forgotten some things your unconscious mind remembers. It's important for our purposes if your unconscious remembers to forget the things it is supposed to let your unconscious mind remember and that your conscious mind remembers to forget the things that your unconscious mind remembers. And your unconscious mind should remember to remember those things that it is supposed to remember and to forget those things that it is supposed to forget, while your conscious mind remembers to remember the things it is supposed to remember and forgets the things it is supposed to forget.

After a few minutes of such a confusing monologue, the subject usually gives up trying to figure out all the meanings and just "escapes" into trance.

SPLITTING

Splitting is distinguishing between two things or two concepts. The main kind of splitting that is used in most hypnosis, Ericksonian included, is between the "conscious mind" and the "unconscious mind." Now there have been a lot of autopsies done and no one has ever found an unconscious mind or a conscious mind, but that does not mean that as a heuristic concept the division has no utility. It is as if we divide human experience and thinking into two parts — some people might call it "right brain" and "left brain," or the "front of your mind" and the "back of your mind." There can be various words and terms for this division, but the important point here is that a split is made. This split is communicated to the subject in two ways, verbally and nonverbally.

Verbal splitting is perhaps obvious from the examples given so far. In just talking about "conscious mind" and "conscious experience" as distinct from "unconscious mind" and "unconscious experience," the hypnotist makes a verbal distinction for the client. This may be one that the client has made before or it may be a new one for him. It starts to create the context in which this split is a natural division, an obvious split, as implied by the words of the hypnotist.

The split may also be implied by the hypnotist's voice tone and behavior. It is difficult to show all the forms of *nonverbal splitting* with the written word, but on a videotape one might see different body positions or facial expressions associated with each side of the split. In addition, certain voice tones or voice volumes may be used when speaking of each side of the split. When the conscious mind is being discussed or referred to, a certain voice tone is used, and when the unconscious mind is discussed, a different voice tone is used. It is mainly a matter of training to be able to notice and deliberately create these shifts in nonverbal behavior.

The other kinds of splits that are usually made in an Ericksonian induction are splits between externally oriented, here-and-now experience and internally oriented, past or future experience. When those kind of splits are offered initially, there is an emphasis on externally oriented awareness and the here-and-now; as time and the induction go on, there is a shift in emphasis to more internal experience that does not involve the present.

LINKING

As previously discussed, certain voice tones are used to indicate communication to the conscious mind and other voice tones are used for communication to the unconscious mind. This can also be described as a type of *nonverbal linking* (joining together or associating two previously unassociated things or concepts). After a time, a certain voice tone or facial expression will cue the subject that this communication is directed to his conscious mind and another kind of voice tone is directed to the unconscious mind. Therefore, certain voice tones become linked to certain experiences, and after a time a certain voice tone can serve to induce a trance or remind the subject of previous trance experiences.

Verbal linking is when some words are used to associate some experiences with other experiences. The simplest kind of linking involves the mere juxtaposition and association of two experiences or behaviors. For example, "You are sitting in the chair and you can go into trance." The next level of linking, which suggests an even stronger causal connection, is contingent linking, which involves implying that one experience is contingent on another. Examples of contingent linking are, "As you listen to the sound of my voice, you can go into trance," and "The more your conscious mind is distracted, the easier it can be for your unconscious mind to help you go into trance." Examples of an even stronger linkage are, "Listening to the sound of my voice can help you go deeper and deeper into trance," and "Sitting in that chair can help you become more and more relaxed and go more and more deeply into trance."

Another approach to bypassing resistance and reassuring anxious subjects is "incorporating." Incorporating involves verbally including the potential distractions and resistances as part of the trance experience. It might be suggested that the person listen to the sounds outside the room and that those sounds can further trance or be part of the trance experience. It might be suggested that the person can be distracted by his own thoughts or his own concerns about his inability to go into a trance or his worries that he won't go deeply into trance.

INTERSPERSAL

Placing a special emphasis on certain words and phrases is labeled the *interspersal technique* in Erickson's work (see Chapter 3 for another discussion). Essentially, in the interspersal technique nonverbal emphasis is used to indirectly make a suggestion. The subject may not be consciously aware of the nonverbal emphasis, but the idea is that he will notice it at some level, subliminally, and respond to it at some level. For instance, if the hypnotist wanted to give an interspersed suggestion for the subject to lift his hand up to his face, he might say, "Your unconscious can come *up* with a lot of things for you, and you really didn't know it probably, but your unconscious can be very *handy* for you, because it has a lot of knowledge. Now, some of that knowledge, some of the things you might experience in trance could be very *disarming*." The underlined words are emphasized nonverbally. These constitute interspersed suggestions. An Ericksonian induction is usually replete with these kinds of suggestions.

EMPTY WORDS

Another aspect of Ericksonian induction is the abundant use of nonspecific words. These "empty" words (discussed earlier in Chapter 7) lack specific meaning and are open to many interpretations. I sometimes call these "politician words," because politicians want to be heard by a large group of people, but they usually do not want to be pinned down to specific meanings. In traditional counseling training, "concreteness" is emphasized as a skill for therapists to use consistently with clients. Here the emphasis is the exact opposite. The goal is to be as unspecific and nonconcrete as possible, in order to facilitate the subject's making his own meanings from the hypnotist's words. Words like "experience," "unconscious," and so forth are not specified as to time, place, person, thing, or action. Think of how a fairy tale starts, "Long ago, far away, there lived a young boy who possessed a curious object and this is the story of what he did with that object and what he learned." This allows for each person to individualize the story for himself as he is listening or reading. In the same way, the use of these words in a trance induction helps the subject to create his own trance experience by interpreting those very ambiguous, empty words the hypnotist uses. One of the difficulties with a technique like guided fantasy is that the words are often too specific for the subject or listener and may interfere with the subject's experience. An Ericksonian guided fantasy might be, "You can go to a particular place and create a particular experience for yourself and go through that experience in a way that is appropriate for you," rather than the very specific, "Now you find yourself in the woods and you're looking up at the trees and you see the light coming down through the trees." Some people will follow along very well with such a guided fantasy, but some people will be lost. Either they won't be able to visualize, or they will feel that they aren't doing it right, or they will be constructing some aspects of the experience that are different from your description of it.

Another effect of these empty words is that the listener focuses more internally in order to make sense of these vague and sometimes confusing utterances.

SUMMARY

Each of these elements by itself may not be sufficient to induce a trance, but put together they create a powerful context that makes it likely the subject will enter a trance. And, of course, the elements that have been separated here are mixed together in practice. In addition, it should be noted that in Erickson's work, induction and treatment were rather inextricably bound. Already during the induction, Erickson was seeding ideas and starting his therapeutic interventions.

10. Frameworks of Erickson's Therapy and Hypnosis

Various students of Erickson have presented his approaches and techniques in systematic, coherent frameworks, in order to make the work more accessible to others. In this chapter, the major frameworks of Erickson's work are summarized. The material is limited to those frameworks which deal with Erickson's hypnosis and/or therapy as a whole. Since each framework has many more details and aspects than can be included here, only a distillation of the essential elements from each is listed. Where the name of the element is not self-explanatory, an explanation or definition is included.

For the most part the frameworks are covered chronologically, with the earliest models being summarized first, except when one person has two or more frameworks from different time periods. For convenience, the models of the same person from different times are summarized in the same section.

HALEY'S FRAMEWORKS

Haley has proposed several different frameworks for Erickson's work at several different times. The different frameworks are not contradictory, just different.

In his first book (1963), Haley listed several elements in Erickson's work. He wrote that Erickson's work could be characterized as directive. The therapist was to get the patient to *do* something. Often the therapist would direct the patient

131

to behave in the symptomatic way with some addition. The therapist used positive redefinition and accepted the patient's behavior to insure cooperation and to facilitate therapy. The directives utilized the patient's assets and personality factors. Implication was often used to indirectly elicit behavior from the patient. The goal of therapy was arranging or changing the environment for symptomatic behavior.

In 1967, in his commentary on Erickson's work in the afterword to his collection of Erickson's papers, Haley detailed several elements that are involved in Erickson's work. These include:

1) *The therapeutic posture*. The therapist must incorporate and modify techniques to express his/her individual personality; therapist must also modify techniques to deal with unique, individual patients.

2) *Expectation of change*. The therapist expects that change is not only possible, but inevitable.

3) *Emphasis on the positive*. Normal behavior and growth are the process of living and psychopathology an interference with that process. The unconscious is a positive aspect of humans, not a cauldron of repressed, primal urges and conflicts. Patient's defects become assets in Erickson's eyes.

4) *Accepting what the patient offers*. This includes symptoms, pessimism, resistance, rigid ideas, and delusions.

5) *Emphasis on the range of possibilities*. Possibilities for the therapist in approaching the patient; possibilities for the patient to behave and to view things differently.

6) *Willingness to take responsibility*. The therapist must be willing to take responsibility and make decisions for people if it is necessary; each case is handled individually as to how much responsibility the therapist needs to take.

7) *Blocking off symptomatic behavior.* The therapist is not concerned with the "roots" of symptomatic behavior, he or she just views it as a malfunctioning to be corrected. To this end, he might block the symptomatic behavior either by relabeling the behavior, by taking it over and changing it under direction, or by providing an ordeal which makes it difficult to continue the symptomatic behavior.

8) *Change occurs in relation to the therapist.* The therapist creates an intense relationship and then uses that relationship to get the person to cooperate or therapeutically rebel or prove the therapist wrong.

9) *Use of anecdotes.* Analogies, stories, anecdotes or jokes are used to peg ideas or to make a previously unacceptable possibility acceptable.

10) *Willingness to release patients.* Once the particular symptom is resolved, the patient is released from treatment. No attempt is made to resolve all present or future difficulties.

11) *Premises of Erickson's approach:*
   a) The focus is on the present.
   b) The focus is on interactions.
   c) Symptoms are communications.
   d) Awareness/insight is unnecessary for change.
   e) The cause of change (and the continuance of that change) is the rearranging of the patient's situation.

In 1973, Haley offered yet another framework for Erickson's work. He examined Erickson's work through the framework of the family life cycle. He characterized Erickson's approach as strategic. He also listed the elements of Erickson's work as follows:

1) Encouraging resistance.
2) Encouraging a response by frustrating it.

3) Encouraging a relapse.
4) Providing a worse alternative.
5) Amplifying a deviation from the usual.
6) Using "hypnotic" skills and communication devices in nonhypnotic therapy, including:
   a) Amnesia and the control of information.
   b) Seeding ideas.
   c) The use of space and position.
   d) Awakening and disengagement.
7) Causing change by communicating in metaphor.

According to Haley, Erickson rarely strived for insight about unconscious processes, interpersonal difficulties, transference or motivations. His therapy was based upon the interpersonal impact of the therapist outside the patient's awareness and included directives that cause changes in behavior.

BEAHRS' FRAMEWORK

Beahrs, in his paper on Erickson's "hypnotic psychotherapy" (1971), provides a framework which includes basic orientations, hypnotic techniques, and therapeutic techniques.

According to Beahrs, the orientations that are present in Erickson's work are:

1) Present or future time orientation.
2) The recognition, acceptance, and participation by the therapist of all levels of the patient's behavior and communication.
3) Indirectness.
4) Manipulation (for the patient's benefit, not for the therapist's pleasure).
5) Versatility.

In this framework there are three types of inductions—"standard" inductions, interspersal techniques, and the surprise technique.

Erickson's *standard inductions* are characterized by an experiential orientation, i.e., they elicit and utilize the patient's internal experience as the induction content. Indirectness is also a characteristic of his inductions. The approach is designed to elicit unconscious responses. Erickson would increase expectancy by inhibiting responses and pauses and hesitations. He would also validate the subject's response (however minimal) by thanking the subject for the response.

Beahrs includes several items in the *interspersal techniques* category, making it broader than Erickson's use of the term. Techniques included here include:

1) Standard induction interspersed with small talk, which is used when no specific problems are in evidence.
2) Utilization techniques, in which the resistances which present obstacles to both hypnosis and therapy are encouraged.
3) The confusion technique, in which the patient is given a set of overwhelmingly illogical statements until he gives up trying to follow and goes into trance. This technique is used for very resistant, obsessive-compulsive intellectualizers.
4) The interspersal technique proper, as Erickson defined it, when suggestions are interspersed in the midst of discussions, dictation, etc.

The *surprise technique* is effected by the therapist offering rapid and unexpected communication or behavior followed by or incorporating a suggestion.

Beahrs lists several general principles that characterize Erickson's therapeutic approaches:

1) The therapist attends to the patient's communication at all levels.
2) The therapist meets the patient at his level.
3) The therapist modifies the patient's behavior, thereby achieving control.
4) The therapist manipulates the patient so his behavior will change from within to be more acceptable to himself or others.
5) New mental patterns should be such as to exclude or displace earlier undesirable ones, and must be compatible with the patient's basic personality structure.
6) One must work with the unconscious, which is viewed as a positive resource rather than a negative cauldron of suppressed primitive urges and conflicts.
7) The chief goal of therapy is not abreaction or uncovering, but coordination between conscious and unconscious functioning.

Beahrs finally looks at Erickson's varied techniques of therapy. For instance he used *behavioral techniques,* such as task assignments, in order to affect conditioning and desensitization. On the other hand, *deep, or uncovering, techniques,* for example automatic writing and drawing, were used to gain access to unconscious material. Indirectness, as well as controlled amnesia to limit the rate of the insight, are essential in uncovering.

Beahrs considers *displacement of cathexis* to be the most significant of Erickson's contributions. In this approach, the patient is guided to transfer psychic energy from the original symptom or conflict to other areas. Sometimes just developing rapport or training the patient in hypnosis will effect such a displacement, as the conflictual energy will divert into the healthy therapeutic relationship and then generalize to other relationships (or, in the case of hypnosis, the energy will transfer to the newly developed hypnotic skills).

The innovative techniques which Erickson used to effect this displacement of cathexis were:

1) Symptom substitution, in which a new symptom that is easier to change or to live with is installed in place of the old.
2) Symptom transformation, which involves redirecting the underlying anxiety or conflict to a new object.
3) Time falsification, either of the past (in which the cathexis is displaced to a newly constructed relationship or experience in the past) or of the future (in which the patient constructs his own fantasy of how his cure will be obtained and the energy is displaced onto this projection).

ROSSI'S FRAMEWORK

Rossi, in three books he coauthored with Erickson (Erickson, Rossi, & Rossi, 1976; Erickson & Rossi, 1979; Erickson & Rossi, 1981), offered analyses and models of Erickson's work.

Two major aspects of Erickson's work are presented as (1) the indirect forms of suggestion, and (2) the utilization approach.

Included in the category of *indirect suggestion* are:

1) *The interspersal approach:*
   a) *Indirect associative focusing.* Mentioning topics (without specifically directing them towards the patient) to initiate associational processes related to those topics.
   b) *Indirect ideodynamic focusing.* Providing examples of responses to prime the patient to respond in the same way.

    c) *Interspersal technique.* Emphasizing certain words or phrases within a conversation or sentence.

2) *Truisms utilizing ideodynamic processes.* Eliciting responses in the motor, sensory-perceptual, affective, and cognitive realms by making a simple statement about that particular experience or behavior.

3) *Truisms utilizing time.* Stating the fact that the desired experience or behavior will occur at some time in the future.

4) *Not knowing, not doing.* Suggestions for allowing, rather than making things happen.

5) *Open-ended suggestions.* Offering a variety of possible responses and validating all as hypnotic responses.

6) *Covering all possibilities of a class of responses.* Restricting the range of possible responses, but accepting and validating all possibilities within that range.

7) *Questions that facilitate new response possibilities:*
    a) *Questions to focus associations.*
    b) *Questions for trance induction by association.*
    c) *Questions facilitating therapeutic responsiveness.*

8) *Compound suggestions.* Usually a truism and a suggestion connected by a conjunction (e.g., "and"):
    a) *The yes set.* Asking a patient various questions to which the answer is "yes" or making observations with which the patient would agree sets up a positive response tendency or set.
    b) *Contingent suggestions.* Linking the suggested response to some already occurring or upcoming behavior or experience.
    c) *Apposition of opposites.* Juxtaposing opposite concepts or experiences.
    d) *The negative.* Juxtaposing the positive with the negative.
    e) *Shock and surprise.* Saying something shocking, provocative or surprising, pausing, then defusing

the situation by completing the sentence to modify the meaning.

9) *Implication.* The therapist structures and directs the patient's associative processes by voice dynamics and language:

   a) The implied directive has three parts: (i) a time-binding introduction; (ii) the implied (or assumed) suggestion; and (iii) a behavioral response to signal when the implied suggestion has been carried out.

10) *Binds.* Offers a free, conscious choice of two or more alternatives; any choice leads behavior in the desired direction.

11) *Double binds.* Offers possibilities of behavior outside the patient's usual range of conscious choice and control:

   a) *Time double bind.*
   b) *Conscious-unconscious double bind.*
   c) *Double dissociation double bind.*
   d) *Reverse set double bind.*
   e) *Non-sequitur double bind.*

12) *Multiple level communication:*

   a) *Stories.*
   b) *Puns.*
   c) *Jokes.*
   d) *Riddles.*
   e) *Folk language.*
   f) *Analogies.*
   g) *Symbols.*

The *utilization approach* is defined as accepting all responses, behavior and ideas as valid and using them to further therapeutic goals. Included in this category are:

1) Accepting and utilizing the patient's manifest behavior.
2) Utilizing the patient's inner realities.

3) Utilizing the patient's resistances:
   a) Displacing and discharging resistance. Eliciting the resistance and diverting it away from the therapy situation.
4) Utilizing the patient's negative affects and confusion.
5) Utilizing the patient's symptoms.

BANDLER AND
GRINDER'S FRAMEWORKS

Richard Bandler and John Grinder have published several frameworks dealing with hypnosis, but here we will deal only with those that are attempts to describe what Erickson did when inducing a trance. In their first published work on Erickson's hypnotic patterns and techniques (Bandler & Grinder, 1975), they delineated a mainly linguistic model for inducing a trance. Almost a mirror (opposite) image of their earlier linguistic model to assist therapists to challenge missing or distorted aspects of a client's world view or verbal reports in therapy (the "Meta Model"), this model is called the "Milton Model."

The Milton Model

The overall pattern of Erickson's hypnotic work, according to this framework, is pacing (matching, accepting, and utilizing the client's experiences and behavior) and leading (assisting the client to gain access to personal resources, to build other experiences or to experience things in a way different from usual). Verbal pacing initially consists of describing to the client his ongoing observable behavior, being careful to stay with sensory-based descriptions of behavior that is occurring. Next the hypnotist starts to describe the client's ongoing, non-observable experience, using these linguistic categories; linguistic causal modeling processes; transderivational phenomena; ambiguity; lesser included structures; and derived meanings.

Linguistic causal modeling is used to tie the sensory-based descriptions to other statements, requests and suggestions of the hypnotist. There are three levels of linguistic causal linkage:

1) *Conjunction.* This involves the use of the connectives "and," "but," etc.
2) *Implied causatives.* This is the use of the connectives "as," "while," "during," "before," "after," etc.
3) *Cause-effect.* This occurs when the hypnotist uses predicates which claim a necessary connection between the portions of experience (e.g., "make," "cause," "require," etc.).

These categories claim or imply a linkage between the present (observed) behavior and the desired experience. Each level implies progressively more linkage and causality.

Transderivational search is the name Bandler and Grinder give to that internal search that a client must do in order to make sense of utterances by the therapist that may have various meanings. In Erickson's hypnotic work, language forms that maximize this process are used to facilitate the induction of trance, the accessing of resources, and the client's active involvement in the hypnotic procedure. The several categories included here are:

1) *Generalized referential index.* These are nouns which do not refer to any specific person, place, thing or time, e.g., " . . . some interesting ideas from someone from another time. . . . "
2) *Selectional restriction.* Using language that syntactically makes sense, but which violates basic cultural/personal understandings, e.g., "The rock yelled at me."
3) *Deletion.* Leaving out the subject (actor) or object (acted upon) in a sentence or phrase, e.g., " . . . and learning . . . and really beginning to wonder. . . . "

4) *Nominalization.* A process (action) word that is used as a noun (thing). This includes elements of deletion and generalized referential index, e.g., " . . . the comforts and understandings. . . . "
5) *Unspecified verbs.* Using a verb that does not specify the action to be performed, e.g., " . . . I'm going to ask you to do something."

There are various types of *ambiguity* in Erickson's work:

1) *Phonological ambiguity.* Puns and homonyms, e.g., "Hand levitation can be a disarming phenomenon."
2) *Syntactic ambiguity.* It is not clear whether the word is being used as one form or another, as in "Hypnotizing hypnotists can be tricky."
3) *Scope ambiguity.* It is not clear when the previous reference ends, e.g., "I can see that you are sitting in a chair and going into a trance . . . can be an interesting experience. . . . "
4) *Punctuation ambiguity.* It is not clear where one sentence ends and the other begins, e.g., "I see you are wearing a watch very carefully that arm and hand."

The category of *lesser included structures* includes:

1) *Embedded questions.* The hypnotist asks a question without really asking, e.g., "I'm wondering if you can really begin to sense the changes."
2) *Embedded commands.* This involves indirectly telling the person to do something without making it an obvious order or demand, e.g., "I think it would be very interesting for you to just relax and go into trance."
3) *Quotes.* Reporting what was said in another setting in order to give the person in front of you the same message, e.g., "Then I told her, 'Just relax and go into a trance.'"

4) *Analogical marking.* This is the technique in which certain parts of a communication are emphasized or marked off analogically to give a separate message within the larger message.

Derived meanings are those which are not stated directly but implied by what the hypnotist says.

1) *Presuppositions.* The structure of the verbalization presumes that something is the case, e.g., "I wonder whether you are aware just how deeply you are in trance."

2) *Conversational postulates.* These are "polite commands" used by most people in daily life to ask for something indirectly. Instead of ordering, "Close the door," one says, "Can you close the door?" or "Is the door open?" or "You can close the door."

Other Conceptions

In various writings and other materials, Bandler and Grinder have developed their own model (called Neurolinguistic Programming) and applied it to hypnosis, but here only those aspects of their work which describe Erickson's work will be considered.

The notion that experience is made up of sensory-based elements of current external or past internal perceptions and representations is the cornerstone of many of the further conceptions offered in this framework. At any given time, a person is experiencing some aspect of what is called a 4-tuple, made up of four sensory elements (visual, auditory, kinesthetic, and gustatory/olfactory). These may be sense data either attended to in the present or represented from the past. What the person attends to is called his representational system. All other aspects of the experience are out of awareness ("unconscious") and accessing those into consciousness is one way to bring about an altered state of consciousness. The sensory process that is used to access experience or memories into consciousness is called the lead system. By utilizing or by-passing one or more of these sensory elements, various therapeutic and hypnotic goals can be accomplished.

The other conception of relevance here is the notion of anchoring. Anchoring is a verbal or nonverbal cue or association with some particular experience. It is used to evoke and alter the client's experience to facilitate therapeutic goals.

Finally, Grinder, DeLozier, and Bandler (1977) offer a sequencing of Erickson's hypnotic work:

1) Accessing and anchoring of experiences.
2) Polarity pacing.
3) Dissociation.
4) Metaphor/meta-instructions.
5) Creation of a reference experience.
6) Testing effectiveness of the work.

GORDON AND
MEYERS-ANDERSON'S FRAMEWORK

David Gordon and Maribeth Meyers-Anderson (1981) offer several algorithms (explicit step-by-step instructions) for describing and reproducing Erickson's therapeutic, rather than strictly hypnotic, work.

They divide the major types of interventions into (1) reference frame interventions, and (2) behavioral interventions. They offer three generalizations about Erickson's basic orientation in therapy:

1) The importance of flexibility of both the client and the therapist.
2) The importance of humor.
3) The future orientation.

In order to gain rapport, they give the three types of "pacing" which are important for the therapist to use: "content," "behavioral," and "cultural." The therapist matches the client's model of the world in each of these areas to develop and maintain rapport.

Under the rubric of *reference frame interventions* (which might also be called reframing), there are three categories, with their corresponding algorithms. The first is called "sorting for assets." It is used when an individual has some behavior or characteristic which is undesirable in his view, but would be difficult or impossible to change. The formula for this intervention is as follows:

1) Identify the cause-effect relationship between the undesired behavior/characteristic and the client's goal.
2) Identify some highly valued desired state or criterion to which the unwanted behavior/characteristic is (or could be) connected.
3) Pace your client's experience by explicitly stating your understanding of what he or she identifies as being the cause and effect of his or her problem situation.
4) Get the individual to commit him or herself to defending his/her present perspective.
5) Make explicit the cause-effect relationship between the client's presently unwanted behavior/characteristic and the highly valued desired state you have identified as being within his or her model of the world.

The second category of reference frame interventions is called "sorting for big liabilities." This is used when it is possible and desirable for the client to change his behavior, but his frame of reference provides him with a rationale that makes such inappropriate behavior acceptable. In such a case the formula provided is:

1) Identify for yourself the pattern of behavior to be changed, making sure that it can be changed AND that it is useful to do so.
2) Identify within your client's model of the world some HIGHLY VALUED criterion, behavior, circumstance, or outcome that is or could be described as being jeopardized by his inappropriate behavior.
3) Pace and enhance your client's security in his acceptance of his present perspective in relation to the inappropriate behavior.
4) Make "explicit" to your client the cause-effect relationship between his present behavior and the jeopardy it creates for what you have identified as being of great importance to him.

The last category of reference frame intervention is called "sorting for relevance." In this pattern, the therapist arranges an experience that naturally generates the desired change in perspective that would lead to the new behavior, rather than explicitly providing that new perspective. The formula for this pattern is:

1) Identify for yourself what change in perspective would be most useful for your client (a change either to seeing a former liability as an asset or to seeing a former acceptable behavior as undesirable).
2) Generate an experience that would NATURALLY lead to the acquisition of that perspective.
3) Maintaining a rapport at all times, assist your client in accessing that experience either through external behavior in the real world or vicariously through the utilization of internal representations.

Behavioral interventions begin with the distinction between the content and patterns of behavior. The content includes specific pieces of behavior involved and the pattern is a sequence of behavior characteristic of some particular context. Next are several premises upon which Erickson's behavioral interventions are based:

1) Because people's behaviors are patterned, any change in that pattern will result in new interactions and experiences.
2) Patterns of behavior are soon perpetuated by the corresponding chains of environmental feedback created by those new behaviors.
3) It is unnecessary to delve into the ontogeny of a problem in order to effect a profound and lasting change.
4) There is a correspondence between one's model of the world and behavior such that altering one's behavior has a direct impact on the individual's experience and generalizations.

Three formulas are given for behavioral interventions. The first is to effect changes in inappropriate behavior through behavioral interventions. The sequence for this pattern is:

1) Explicitly identify for yourself the outcome for your client in terms of what behavior and/or interactions are needed within the problem context.
2) Identify for yourself a situation which NATURALLY (normally) results in anyone's engaging in such behavior or interactions.
3) Utilize rapport and, if necessary, changes in frames of reference in order to inject your client into that situation.

The next algorithm is used for altering limiting frames through behavioral interventions:

1) Specify for yourself what would constitute appropriate behavior within the problem context and what

change in perspective would naturally produce that behavior.

2) Identify for yourself what real world experience would naturally install in almost any individual the belief or perspective you want your client to have.

3) Identify for yourself what behavior you could engage your client in that would naturally foment the previously identified experience AND, if possible, utilize as a catalyst that characteristic or behavior that the client identifies as being the "cause" of the problem.

4) Utilize rapport and any necessary reference frame shifts to motivate your client to engage in the behavior.

The last behavior pattern Gordon and Meyers-Anderson specify is for the person who is compulsively doing some habitual behavior that he or she would like to stop:

1) Accept the client's unwanted behavior.

2) Attach as a contingent to it some additional piece of behavior that will eventually prove decisively burdensome.

OMER'S FRAMEWORK

In an article published in 1982, Haim Omer offered a model of Erickson's therapeutic techniques. He divides the strategic functions in Erickson's therapy into three categories: (1) mobilization of change-promoting factors; (2) creation of boundaries facilitating change, and (3) symptom modification and decontextualization.

In the category of *mobilization of change-promoting forces* are:

1) *Capitalizing on misery.* Erickson allows or encourages the patient's pessimism to reach low ebb and then starts treatment.

2) *The pressure cooker technique.* Building naturally growing urges to change and then blocking the patient's
normal outlets.
3) *The Hitchcock ploy.* Erickson entices the patient's curiosity on a vital issue and then delays the satisfaction
of that curiosity.

Creation of boundaries facilitating change breaks time up
into distinct phases by providing a "change" milestone as a
rite of passage. This category includes:

1) *The dramatic overture.* Erickson begins treatment with
exaggerated flourish and fanfare.
2) *Precommitment.* The patient agrees to abide by the
therapist's order, no matter what.
3) *Achieving closure.* Dramatic or clear indications for the
termination of the therapy are provided.
4) *The therapeutic ordeal.* A rite of passage, with a clear
break from the previous situation, an extreme inten-
sification of therapeutic pressure leading to an ordeal,
and a gradual assumption of the new normal life role.

Symptom modification involves encouraging the symptom
with immediate modifications of the symptom itself. It usually
proceeds by minimal steps. Decontextualization (which involves far-reaching modifications of the symptom's context)
is accompanied by great leaps or reversals. Included in these
categories are:

1) *Gradual symptom modification.* Slight changes in the
symptom are gradually introduced.
2) *The divide and rule technique.* A symptom is broken
into successive stages and the therapist either blocks
the progression from one stage to another or mixes up
their normal order.
3) *Modifying the spatial context.* Changing the location
in which the symptom occurs.

4) *Modifying the interpersonal context.* Reversing or altering the interactions surrounding and supporting the symptom.

5) *Modifying the affective context.* Reversing or altering the feelings associated with the symptom.

6) *Modifying the cognitive context.* Reframing, reconnoting, or redefining the symptom.

LANKTONS' FRAMEWORK

In their 1983 book, Steve and Carol Lankton offer a model that both describes Erickson's work and offers further conceptions that the Lanktons have developed in their work. What will be described here are only those aspects of their framework that deal with descriptions of Erickson's work.

First they offer three features that typify an Ericksonian approach:

1) *Indirection.* The use of indirect suggestion, binds, metaphor and resource retrieval.

2) *Conscious/unconscious dissociation.* Multiple level communication, interspersal, double binds and multiple embedded metaphors.

3) *Utilization of the client's behavior.* Paradox, behavioral matching, naturalistic induction, symptom prescription and strategic use of trance phenomena.

Next are the principles underlying Erickson's work:

1) People operate out of their internal maps and not out of sensory experience.

2) People make the best choice for themselves at any given moment.

3) The explanation, theory, or metaphor used to relate facts about a person is not the person.

4) Respect all messages from the client.

5) Teach choice; never attempt to take choice away.
6) The resources the client needs lie within his or her own personal history.
7) Meet the client at his or her model of the world.
8) The person with the most flexibility or choice will be the controlling element in the system.
9) A person can't not communicate.
10) If it's hard work, reduce it down.
11) Outcomes are determined at the psychological level.

The flow of induction is delineated as:

1) Orient to trance.
2) Fixate attention and rapport.
3) Create conscious/unconscious dissociation.
4) Ratify and deepen the trance state
5) Establish a learning frame or learning set.
6) Utilize trance state and phenomena for clinical goals.
7) Reorient to waking state.

Trance phenomena are used strategically to retrieve resources. There are four ways given to elicit trance phenomena:

1) Direct suggestions.
2) Indirect suggestions.
3) Anecdotes and metaphors.
4) Structured amnesia.

The model of metaphor given by the Lanktons includes several elements and is structured to elicit amnesia for the direct work that is done within the session. The phases of this model, called "multiple embedded metaphor" are:

1) Induction.
2) Matching metaphor.
3) Metaphor to retrieve resources.

4) Direct work on core issue.
5) Linking resources to the social network.
6) End matching metaphor.
7) Reorient to waking state.

LUSTIG'S FRAMEWORK

Herbert Lustig has provided what is surely the most parsimonious model of Erickson's work. He introduced this framework, called "The Mastery Model," in a videotape entitled "A Primer of Ericksonian Psychotherapy" (1984).

The Mastery Model has four steps:

1) To LEARN or remember some skill or experience.
2) To PRACTICE using that skill or accessing that memory.
3) To MASTER using that skill.
4) To EXPAND beyond the practice situation and the session to future situations where the skill is needed.

HAVENS' FRAMEWORK

Ronald Havens was disappointed that Erickson died before he had a chance to go and study with him. To compensate in part for that disappointment, he decided to take a sabbatical from his university teaching position and use the time to intensively study Erickson's work. He read all the literature, listened to all the audiotapes available at that time (1980–1981), and wrote down quotations from Erickson that seemed to be significant (Havens, 1981). What emerged from that study was a natural organization of Erickson's approach and philosophy, entitled *The Wisdom of Milton H. Erickson* (Havens, 1984).

Havens' book organizes Erickson's philosophy under a number of headings and topics.

1) *Objective observation yields wisdom.* Erickson stressed using your senses to observe what your patients and other people are doing and saying, as well as yourself. He recommended "objective" observation, which means observing without adding your own interpretations or preconceptions. Areas for observation he focused on included breathing patterns, one's own body, the variable and idiosyncratic meaning of words, nonverbal communication, physiological patterns, behavioral patterns, and cultural differences.

2) *The conscious mind.* Erickson did not share most psychodynamic practitioners' view that the unconscious material should be interpreted to the conscious mind. He viewed conscious frames of reference as often rigid and non-objective. There are, however, always many alternative conscious sets and "personalities."

3) *The unconscious mind.* Erickson viewed the unconscious as a real entity, with its own separate abilities. The unconscious is a storehouse of unknown and latent potentials; it is brilliant, aware, literal and childlike; it is a source of emotions; and it is universal.

4) *What is abnormal?* Havens summarized Erickson's view: "Any behavior that does not serve a useful and meaningful goal for the person, that is at variance with that individual's personality, or that actually interferes with that person's ability to attain reasonable personal goals is abnormal or undesirable" (Havens, 1984, p. 87). Abnormality can arise from conscious limitations and rigidities of behavior and thinking or from repression.

5) *The goal of psychotherapy.* Here Havens offers five statements on Erickson's goals and principles of psychotherapy:
   a) Focus on the possible, not on perfection.

      b) Focus on the future, not on the past.

      c) Objectivity cures.

      d) Behavior and experiences can initiate therapeutic reorganization.

      e) Patients can and must do the therapy.

6) *Creating a psychotherapeutic climate.* The following are tasks for the therapist and facts about patients for therapists to consider:

      a) Therapists provide therapeutic climates.

      b) Therapists provide motivation.

      c) Therapists solicit trust and motivation.

      d) Therapists recognize and accept each patient's limitations.

      e) Patients are ambivalent about therapy.

      f) Patients are unreliable sources, so therapists must decipher what they say.

      g) Therapists must acknowledge the patient's reality.

      h) Therapists protect and give freedom to patients.

      i) The patient's welfare should be the major concern of the therapist.

7) *Initiating therapeutic change.* Patients are unique, so therapists should use whatever they present rather than having some preconceived notions and approaches. This includes using the patient's desires and expectations, language, emotions, resistance, and symptoms. The therapist should rely on his own observations, rather than on some theory he learned from a book.

8) *Understanding hypnosis.* Trance is focused attention; during trance reality is less important and attention is turned inward. Hypnosis facilitates rapport and responsiveness. Hypnosis does not create new abilities, but offers access to unused potentials, which are accessed through revivification of patients' previous experiences. Hypnotized subjects are not automa-

tons; they can and do respond in a variety of ways. Since deep trance involves the unconscious, patients are literal and childlike when in deep trance.

9) *Inducing hypnosis.* Anyone can be hypnotized. Hypnosis requires the right atmosphere and eliciting cooperation from the subject, so the hypnotist's language and approach must be tailored to use whatever the subject presents. The hypnotist must keep his role and goal in mind, which is to fixate attention and direct it away from external reality towards inner experience.

10) *Utilizing hypnosis therapeutically.* Hypnosis is only a tool. It increases access to potentials, facilitates learning and overcomes conscious limitations. Hypnosis allows unconscious therapy; it is best to let psychotherapy remain out of conscious awareness. Trance phenomena, such as ideomotor responses, time distortion, age regression, dissociation, amnesia, etc., can be used therapeutically.

ZEIG'S FRAMEWORK

Zeig (1985) provides a framework for Erickson's "utilization" approach. Important issues in this approach are:

1) Identify the resource (unaccessed strengths) in the patient.
2) Diagnose the patient's values, i.e., what the patient likes and dislikes (which can also be resources).
3) Develop the resource by utilizing the patient's values.
4) Connect the developed resource to the problem, either directly or indirectly.
5) Get people to do things, usually in small steps, accessing trust, rapport and motivation, and guiding responsiveness throughout the process.

6) Any behavior, even resistance, and any aspect of the context can be accepted and utilized therapeutically.
7) Drama can be used to enhance responsiveness to directives.
8) Seeding ideas prior to presenting them primes responsive behavior.
9) Timing is crucial. The process of therapy involves pacing, disrupting, and patterning. Resistance often results from inadequate attention to these processes.
10) The therapist and the patient must have an expectant attitude.
11) Test the effectiveness of the intervention in the office or from follow-up contacts.

CLOSING REMARKS

In this chapter and, indeed, this whole book, I have attempted to summarize the current state of available frameworks for understanding and reproducing the hypnotic and psychotherapeutic work of Milton H. Erickson. It is hoped that such a summary will help both to make Erickson's work more accessible and to point to future directions in the development of new frameworks.

Further
Resources

Further

Resources

Bibliography of Ericksonian Approaches and Techniques

BOOKS BY MILTON H. ERICKSON, M.D.

Collected Papers

Haley, Jay. *Advanced techniques of hypnosis and therapy: Selected papers of Milton H. Erickson, M.D.* New York: Grune and Stratton, 1967.

> This was the first effort to compile Erickson's major papers on hypnosis and therapy. It also contains a biographical introduction and discussion of Erickson's work by Haley, Erickson's longtime student and popularizer. All of this material, with the exception of Haley's writing, is included in the *Collected Papers* (see next entry).

Rossi, Ernest L. *The collected papers of Milton Erickson on hypnosis.* New York: Irvington, 1980.

> This four-volume work includes all of Erickson's published papers on hypnosis and therapy, some previously unpublished material and a few papers by Erickson's collaborators (Rossi, Elizabeth Erickson, Jeff Zeig and others). Volume 1 includes material on "The Nature of Hypnosis and Suggestion," Volume 2 is about "Hypnotic Alteration of Sensory, Perceptual and Psychophysiological Processes," Volume 3 covers "Hypnotic Investigation of Psychodynamic Processes," and Volume 4 is on "Innovative Hypnotherapy."

Co-authored Books

Cooper, Linn and Erickson, Milton H. *Time distortion in hypnosis.* New York: Irvington, 1982 (reissued).

> The results of Erickson and Cooper's experimental and clinical work in this area. Much of this material is included in the *Collected Papers.*

Erickson, Milton, H., Hershman, Seymour, and Secter, Irving I. *The practical application of medical and dental hypnosis*. Chicago: Seminars on Hypnosis Publishing Co., 1981 (reissued).

This book was compiled primarily from transcripts of workshops for medical, psychological and dental professionals given by the authors during the late 1950s.

Erickson, Milton, H., Rossi, Ernest L., and Rossi, Sheila I. *Hypnotic realities: The induction of clinical hypnosis and forms of indirect suggestion*. New York: Irvington, 1976.

The first book in a series of three co-authored by Erickson and Rossi. Gives an overall model for Erickson's hypnotic approaches. Contains numerous discussions and commentaries on transcripts of inductions. Accompanied by an audiocassette of Erickson doing two trance inductions with the same subject.

Erickson, Milton H. and Rossi, Ernest L. *Hypnotherapy: An exploratory casebook*. New York: Irvington, 1979.

The second book in the series. This volume deals extensively with hypnotic therapy, utilizing numerous case examples and transcripts. A tape of a therapy session conducted by Erickson with a man with phantom limb pain and his wife with tinnitus accompanies this book.

Erickson, Milton H. and Rossi, Ernest L. *Experiencing hypnosis: Therapeutic approaches to altered states*. New York: Irvington, 1981.

The third book in the series, containing a transcript of a lecture on hypnosis in psychiatry by Erickson and discussion of various therapeutic techniques and approaches. Includes a detailed description of Erickson's famous nonverbal arm catalepsy induction technique. Two audiocassettes (of the lecture mentioned above) accompany this book.

BOOKS EDITED BY OTHERS
(PRIMARILY CONSISTING OF ERICKSON'S MATERIAL)

Haley, Jay. *Conversations with Milton H. Erickson, M.D. Volume 1: Changing individuals; Volume 2: Changing couples; Volume 3: Changing children and families*. New York: Triangle (distributed by Norton), 1985.

These conversations took place mainly in the late 1950s among Erickson, Haley, John Weakland, and occasionally Gregory Bateson. Haley and Weakland were trying to understand Erickson's brief therapy for their research with Bateson's project on communication and for their own clinical work with individuals, couples and families. Reading the books is like reading the transcripts of supervision sessions with some theoretical material and some case discussion. This material was the source for much of the material in *Uncommon therapy*.

Havens, Ronald. *The wisdom of Milton H. Erickson.* New York: Irvington, 1984.

This book is a compilation of quotations from Erickson on various topics relating to therapy and hypnosis. The quotations are organized into sections and what emerges constitutes a natural model for Erickson's therapeutic and hypnotic approaches.

Rosen, Sidney. *My voice will go with you: The teaching tales of Milton H. Erickson.* New York: Norton, 1982.

A collection of some of Erickson's often used teaching stories, some case examples, some personal and family anecdotes, with commentary and organization by Rosen.

Rossi, Ernest L., Ryan, Margaret O., and Sharp, Florence A. *Healing in hypnosis: The seminars, workshops and lectures of Milton H. Erickson, Volume 1.* New York: Irvington, 1983.

This is the first in a projected three to five volume series of transcripts of Erickson's lectures and demonstrations from the 1950s and '60s. This volume also contains a short biography and some pictures of Erickson over the years. It is accompanied by a tape of one of the lectures transcribed in the book.

Rossi, Ernest L. and Ryan, Margaret O. *Life reframing in hypnosis: The seminars, workshops and lectures of Milton H. Erickson, Volume 2.* New York: Irvington, 1985.

This is a continuation of the volume above with more of the same. Included with the book is a tape of Erickson doing hypnotic therapy with a photographer, which is transcribed in the book.

Zeig, Jeffrey K. *A teaching seminar with Milton H. Erickson.* New York: Brunner/Mazel, 1980.

Transcript of a five-day teaching seminar that Erickson gave near the end of his life. It includes a number of anecdotes, some inductions, and dialogues with students. Introductory chapter by Zeig on Erickson's use of anecdotes. Includes a discussion and commentary by Erickson and Zeig on a trance induction which occurred during the seminar. Spotlights Erickson's unique oral teaching ability.

Zeig, Jeffrey K. *Experiencing Erickson: An introduction to the man and his work.* New York: Brunner/Mazel, 1985.

This book contains an overview and introduction to Erickson as a person and as a therapist, as well as transcripts of Erickson's supervision and teaching with Zeig.

BOOKS PRIMARILY ABOUT ERICKSONIAN APPROACHES

Bandler, Richard and Grinder, John. *Patterns of the hypnotic techniques of Milton H. Erickson, M.D. Volume 1.* Cupertino, California: Meta, 1975.

This is a how-to manual for reproducing Erickson's use of language in trance inductions. The model presented is based on transformational grammar and split-brain research.

Dolan, Yvonne. *A path with a heart: Ericksonian utilization with resistant and chronic patients.* New York: Brunner/Mazel, 1985.

This book presents an extension of Ericksonian principles and techniques into work with difficult, multiproblem, long-term patients.

Gordon, David and Meyers-Anderson, Maribeth. *Phoenix: Therapeutic patterns of Milton H. Erickson.* Cupertino, California: Meta, 1981.

An attempt at systematizing and making explicit Erickson's therapeutic (as opposed to strictly hypnotic) work. Uses material from Erickson's teaching seminars to illustrate the principles discussed.

Grinder, John, DeLozier, Judith, and Bandler, Richard. *Patterns of the hypnotic techniques of Milton H. Erickson, M.D. Volume 2.* Cupertino, California: Meta, 1977.

This second book in the series (see Bandler and Grinder, above) offers conceptions of sensory-based maps, different approaches for congruent and incongruent clients, and other ideas about Erickson's hypnotic work. A transcript of Erickson's work (taken from *The Artistry of Milton Erickson* videotape) is analyzed with reference to the formulations presented in both volumes.

Haley, Jay. *Uncommon therapy: The psychiatric techniques of Milton H. Erickson, M.D.* New York: Norton, 1973.

Contains numerous case examples, discussions with Erickson, commentaries and specific techniques. The book is mainly about Erickson's therapeutic approaches. The material is organized and presented within the family life cycle framework.

Haley, Jay. *Ordeal therapy: Unusual ways to change behavior.* San Francisco: Jossey-Bass, 1984.

This is an extension of the benevolent ordeal therapy Haley learned from Erickson. Some Erickson cases are used, but the majority come from cases Haley supervised or treated himself.

Lankton, Stephen and Lankton, Carol. *The answer within: A clinical framework of Ericksonian hypnotherapy.* New York: Brunner/Mazel, 1983.

Contains case examples from Erickson's and the Lanktons' work embedded in a comprehensive framework to provide clinicians access to Ericksonian approaches to the use of hypnosis in therapy. An audiotape of the Lanktons doing hypnotherapy is available to accompany the volume.

Lankton, Stephen (Editor). *Elements and dimensions of an Ericksonian approach.* New York: Brunner/Mazel, 1985.

This is the first volume in a continuing series of Ericksonian Monographs, sponsored by the Erickson Foundation as a forum for continuing education and information exchange. This volume contains a variety of articles on different applications of Erickson's work. It includes a new article, contributed by Elizabeth Erickson, that is an update of an unpublished Milton Erickson article on certain principles of medical hypnosis.

Overholser, Lee C. *Ericksonian hypnosis: Handbook of clinical practice.* New York: Irvington, 1984.

This is a primer on the induction and therapeutic use of hypnosis using an Ericksonian approach. It includes exercises at the end of each chapter to practice the skills discussed.

Zeig, Jeffrey K. (Editor). *Ericksonian approaches to hypnosis and psychotherapy.* New York: Brunner/Mazel, 1982.

Edited proceedings of the First International Congress on Ericksonian Approaches to Hypnosis and Psychotherapy, which was held in Phoenix in 1980. Includes keynote addresses by Jay Haley and Carl Whitaker and 41 other papers on Erickson and Ericksonian approaches in various areas of social science and medicine.

Zeig, Jeffrey K. (Editor). *Ericksonian psychotherapy. Volume 1: Structures; Volume 2: Clinical applications.* New York: Brunner/Mazel, 1985.

These are the edited proceedings of the Second International Erickson Congress, held in Phoenix in 1983. Keynote and plenary addresses are by Watzlawick, Rossi, Haley and Madanes. Includes a special section by Erickson's family on his childrearing techniques. These volumes are meant to show the development and furthering of Erickson's work in new directions and to show new applications for Erickson's techniques and approaches.

Videotapes of
Milton H. Erickson

The artistry of Milton H. Erickson, M.D. Part I (53 minutes), Part II (51 minutes). $225 each on videocassette or $400 for both; $1000 each on film or $1800 for both. Available from Irvington Publishers and Herbert Lustig, P.O. Box 261, Haverford, PA 19041.

The reverse set in hypnotic induction. One videocassette, 45 minutes. $185 from Irvington Publishers.

Symbolic hypnotherapy. One videocassette. 156 minutes. $200 from The Milton H. Erickson Foundation, 3606 N. 24th St., Phoenix, AZ 85016.

The process of hypnotic induction: A training videotape featuring inductions conducted by Milton H. Erickson in 1964. 120 minutes. $150 from The Milton H. Erickson Foundation.

1958 Milton H. Erickson Hypnotic Induction. 40 minutes. $425 (½" or ¾" formats) from The Family Therapy Institute of Washington, DC, 5850 Hubbard Drive, Rockville, MD 20852.

Audiotapes of Milton H. Erickson

Control of physiological functions by hypnosis/hypnotic approaches to therapy. Four cassettes. Recorded 1952. From The Milton H. Erickson Foundation.

Hypnosis in psychiatry; The Ocean Monarch Lecture. Two cassettes. 120 minutes. From Irvington Publishers. [Accompanies the book *Experiencing hypnosis*.]

The psychodynamics of hypnosis/advanced techniques I: permissive language, ordeal therapy, geometric progressions/advanced techniques II: double binds. Four cassettes. Recorded 1960. From The Milton H. Erickson Foundation. [Includes some demonstrations.]

Advanced psychotherapy. One cassette. 62 minutes. Recorded August 1966. From American Society of Clinical Hypnosis. [Currently unavailable.]

Anxiety and resistance: How to speak to your patients and how to hear them. Three cassettes. 186 minutes. Recorded February 1966. From American Society of Clinical Hypnosis. [Currently unavailable.]

Hypnosis and pain. One cassette. 52 minutes. Recorded July 1965. From American Society of Clinical Hypnosis. [Currently unavailable.]

Recovering traumatic events. One cassette. 67 minutes. Recorded August 1964. From American Society of Clinical Hypnosis. [Currently unavailable.]

General considerations in hypnosis. One cassette. 70 minutes. Recorded July 1965. From American Society of Clinical Hypnosis. [Currently unavailable.]

Healing in hypnosis: A demonstration of trance in everyday life by Milton
H. Erickson. One cassette. 60 minutes. From Irvington Publishers. [Accompanies the book *Healing in hypnosis.*]

SESSIONS AND DEMONSTRATIONS

Life reframing in hypnosis. One cassette. Date unknown. From Irvington
Publishers. [Accompanies the book *Life reframing in hypnosis.*]

Hypnotic realities. One cassette. 60 minutes. From Irvington Publishers.
[Accompanies the book *Hypnotic realities.*]

Hypnotherapy. One cassette. 60 minutes. From Irvington Publishers. [Accompanies the book *Hypnotherapy.*]

Research on Erickson's Approaches and Techniques

Alman, Brian M. (1979). *Consequences of direct and indirect suggestions on success of post-hypnotic behavior.* Unpublished doctoral dissertation, California School of Professional Psychology, San Diego.

Alman, Brian M. and Richard E. Carney (1980). Consequences of direct and indirect suggestions on success of posthypnotic behavior. *American Journal of Clinical Hypnosis,* 23(2): 112–118, October.

Angelos, James Steven (1978). *A comparison of the effects of direct and indirect methods of hypnotic induction on the perception of pain.* Unpublished doctoral dissertation, California School of Professional Psychology, San Diego.

Shulik, A. (1979). *Right- versus left-hemispheric communication styles in hypnotic inductions and the facilitation of hypnotic trance.* Unpublished doctoral dissertation, California School of Professional Psychology, Fresno.

Stone, Jennifer A. and Lundy, Richard M. (1985). Behavioral compliance with direct and indirect body movement suggestions. *Journal of Abnormal Psychology,* 94(3): 256–263, August.

White, D. (1979). *Ericksonian hypnotherapeutic approaches: A case study of the treatment of obesity using indirect forms of suggestion.* Unpublished doctoral dissertation, U.S. International University, San Diego.

Wilson, John Gerald (1974). *The hypnotic relationship: Facilitation and inhibition through indirect procedures.* Unpublished doctoral dissertation, Michigan State University.

An Ericksonian Glossary

Every field has its jargon and Ericksonian therapy is no exception. This glossary is included to help readers who may be unfamiliar with hypnosis or Erickson's names for techniques.

Age regression — A hypnotic technique that involves taking a subject mentally back to some earlier stage of life.

Amnesia — A hypnotic technique that arranges for the subject to forget some or all aspects of a session or some other information.

Analgesia — Hypnotic technique whereby pain is eliminated or reduced.

Anesthesia — Eliminating sensations through hypnosis.

Arm levitation — Hypnotically eliciting an automatic lifting of the subject's hand and arm.

Catalepsy — Rigidity of the limbs or the body induced by trance.

Confusion technique — Using too much detail, non sequiturs, or ambiguous communications to overwhelm the conscious, logical aspects of the person in order to facilitate trance induction or to bypass conscious limitations.

Dissociation — Distinguishing between two experiences or elements by words or actions.

Hand levitation — See arm levitation.

Handshake induction — Erickson's technique of interrupting a handshake to induce a trance and catalepsy of the arm by using ambiguous touches and gazes.

Illusion of alternatives — Giving the patient two or more alternatives, any of which, if chosen, would lead in the desired direction or have the desired result.

Implication — Indirectly suggesting some idea or action to a person.

Indirect suggestion — Any communication technique used to deliver suggestions in an oblique manner. Includes presupposition, interspersal and parallel communication.

Interspersal technique — Devised by Erickson to deliver messages indirectly to patients. The technique involves embedding messages with different nonverbal (such as voice tone shifts, volume shifts, etc.) or verbal aspects (e.g., saying something very clear and straightforward in the midst of a lot of ambiguous and confusing talk) in the communication to the patient.

My friend John technique — Inducing a trance by telling about a previous induction that was done. By including the exact words and intonations while recounting the previous induction, an induction can be done without the subject's awareness.

Naturalistic approach — Using what natural conditions exist within or around the person to induce a trance or accomplish therapy. This approach involves assuming that the patient or subject has everything he needs in order to go into a trance and/or to accomplish the therapeutic goals. The approach also involves using a casual, nonritualized approach to therapy and induction.

Parallel communication — Talking about one thing or area to communicate indirectly about another situation. Includes anecdotes, analogies, jokes, riddles and other metaphorical devices.

Pattern intervention — Wider than pattern interruption, this category includes interrupting a pattern, channeling a pattern, establishing a new pattern, etc. The idea is to alter the pattern in such a way that it is broken or moved in the direction of symptom relief.

Posthypnotic suggestion — A hypnotic technique for directing the subject to perform certain actions or have certain experiences at some time after the trance.

Pseudo-orientation in time — Hypnotically orienting the subject to either the past or the future.

Reframing — Offering a new meaning of a situation, symptom, action, etc.

Surprise technique — Inducing a trance or challenging a patient's frame of reference by shocking the patient with unexpected behavior or communication by the therapist.

Symptom substitution — Giving the patient a new symptom to substitute for the old one, either as a step to resolving the symptom or to provide a symptom that is not so disruptive and painful for the patient.

Symptom transformation — Taking the underlying energy or thinking involved in a symptom and transferring it to another object or direction.

Time distortion — Altering a hypnotic subject's subjective experience of time flow, either stretching it out or contracting it.

Utilization — Using whatever the patient or subject brings to the situation to accomplish trance or therapeutic goals.

References

Bandler, R., & Grinder, J. (1975). *Patterns of the hypnotic techniques of Milton H. Erickson, M.D., Vol. 1*, Cupertino, CA: Meta.
Beahrs, J. (1971). The hypnotic psychotherapy of Milton H. Erickson. *American Journal of Clinical Hypnosis*, 14(2): 73–90, October.
Booth, P. (1984). Personal communication.
Brown, G. S. (1972). *Laws of form*. New York: Bantam.
Camus, A. (1957). *The fall*. New York: Knopf.
Erickson, M. H. (1960). *Advanced techniques I* (audiotape). Phoeniz, AZ: Milton H. Erickson Foundation, Inc.
Erickson, M. H. (1966). *Advanced psychotherapy* (audiotape). Des Plaines, IL: The American Society of Clinical Hypnosis.
Erickson, M. H. (1977). Personal communication (live supervision).
Erickson, M. H. (1979). Brochure for the First International Erickson Congress. Phoenix, Arizona: Milton H. Erickson Foundation.
Erickson, M. H. (1983). Quotation in *NYSEPH Newsletter*, 1(2): 3, February.
Erickson, M., Rossi, E., & Rossi, S. (1976). *Hypnotic realities*. New York: Irvington.
Erickson, M., & Rossi, E. (1979). *Hypnotherapy: An exploratory casebook*. New York: Irvington.
Erickson, M., & Rossi, E. (1981). *Experiencing hypnosis*. New York: Irvington.
Eysenck, H. J. (1957). *Sense and nonsense in psychology*. Middlesex, England: Penguin.
Gordon, D., & Meyers-Anderson, M. (1981). *Phoenix: Therapeutic patterns of Milton H. Erickson*. Cupertino, California: Meta.
Grinder, J., DeLozier, J., & Bandler, R. (1977). *Patterns of the hypnotic techniques of Milton H. Erickson, M.D., Vol. 2*. Cupertino, California: Meta.
Haley, J. (1963). *Strategies of psychotherapy*. New York: Grune & Stratton.
Haley, J. (1973). *Uncommon therapy: The psychiatric techniques of Milton H. Erickson, M.D.* New York: Norton.
Haley, J. (Ed.) (1967). *Advanced techniques of hypnosis and therapy*. New York: Grune & Stratton.
Haley, J. (1982). The contribution to therapy of Milton H. Erickson, M.D.

171

172   *Taproots*

In J. K. Zeig (Ed.), *Ericksonian approaches to hypnosis and psychotherapy* (pp. 5–25). New York: Brunner/Mazel.

Haley, J. (1984). *Ordeal therapy.* San Francisco: Jossey-Bass.

Haley, J. (1985). *Conversations with Milton H. Erickson, M.D.* (3 volumes). New York: Triangle. (Distributed by Norton.)

Havens, R. (1981). Personal communication (letter).

Keeney, B. (1983). *Aesthetics of change.* New York: Guilford.

Keeney, B. (1985). *Mind in therapy: Constructing systemic family therapies.* New York: Basic.

Lankton, S., & Lankton, C. (1983). *The answer within.* New York: Brunner/Mazel.

Lustig, H. (1975). *The Artistry of Milton H. Erickson* (videotape). Ardmore, PA.

Madanes, C. (1981). *Strategic family therapy.* San Francisco: Jossey-Bass.

Madanes, C. (1984). *Behind the one-way mirror.* San Francisco: Jossey-Bass.

O'Hanlon, B. (1982). Splitting and linking: Two generic patterns in Ericksonian therapy. *Journal of Strategic and Systemic Therapies,* 1(4): 21–25, Winter.

O'Hanlon, B., & Wilk, J. (1987). *Shifting contexts: The generation of effective psychotherapy.* New York: Guilford.

Pachter, H. M. (1982). *Magic into science: The story of Paracelsus.* New York: Arden Library.

Postman, N. (1976). *Crazy talk, stupid talk.* New York: Dell.

Rajneesh, B. S. (1978). *Ecstasy—The forgotten language.* Poona, India: Rajneesh Foundation.

Ritterman, M. (1985). Family context, symptom induction and therapeutic counterinduction: Breaking the spell of a dysfunction rapport. In J. K. Zeig (Ed.), *Ericksonian Psychotherapy, Vol. 2: Clinical Applications.* New York: Brunner/Mazel.

Rosen, S. (1982). *My voice will go with you.* New York: Norton.

Rossi, E. L. (Ed.) (1980). *The collected papers of Milton H. Erickson, M.D.* (4 volumes). New York: Irvington.

Rossi, E. L. (1982). Hypnosis and ultradian cycles: A new state(s) theory of hypnosis? *The American Journal of Clinical Hypnosis,* 1: 21–32.

Rossi, E. L. (1985). Altered states of consciousness in everyday life: The ultradian rhythms. In B. Wolman (Ed.), *Handbook of altered states of consciousness.* New York: Van Nostrand.

Rossi, E., & Ryan, M. (1985). *Life reframing in hypnosis.* New York: Irvington.

Rossi, E., Ryan, M., & Sharp, F. (1983). *Healing in hypnosis.* New York: Irvington.

Scheflen, A. E. (1965). Quasi-courting behavior in psychotherapy. *Psychiatry,* 28: 245–257.

Time staff. (1973). Svengali in Arizona, *Time,* October 22.

Watzlawick, P., Weakland, J., & Fisch, R. (1974). *Change: Principles of problem formation and problem resolution.* New York: Norton.
Watzlawick, P. (Ed.) (1984). *The invented reality.* New York: Norton.
Wilk, J. (1985). That reminds me of a story. *Family Therapy Networker,* 9(2): 45–48.
Zeig, J. K. (1980). *A teaching seminar with Milton H. Erickson.* New York: Brunner/Mazel.
Zeig, J. (1981). Personal communication.
Zeig, J. (1982). *Introduction to Ericksonian hypnosis* (audiotape). Phoenix, AZ: Milton H. Erickson Foundation, Inc.
Zeig, J. (1984). Personal communication.
Zeig, J. (1985). *Experiencing Erickson.* New York: Brunner/Mazel.

Index

175